ARSENAL OF
HOPE

TACTICS FOR TAKING ON
PTSD, TOGETHER

JEN SATTERLY
HOLLY LORINCZ

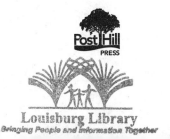

Post Hill
PRESS

Louisburg Library
Bringing People and Information Together

A POST HILL PRESS BOOK
ISBN: 978-1-64293-679-7
ISBN (eBook): 978-1-64293-680-3

Arsenal of Hope:
Tactics for Taking on PTSD, Together

Cover Photo: California National Guardsman hanging out window of train, kissing his wife good-bye, 1950, *Los Angeles Times* Photographic Archives (Collection 1429). Library Special Collections, Charles E. Young Research Library, UCLA

Post Hill Press
New York • Nashville
posthillpress.com

Published in the United States of America
1 2 3 4 5 6 7 8 9 10

DEDICATED TO

My son and daughter, Luke and Claudia,
Never stop being uniquely and amazingly you.

—Jen

ADVANCE PRAISE FOR
ARSENAL OF HOPE

"*Arsenal of Hope* is above all, a love story. *Arsenal of Hope* echoes with the universal truth that resilience is not about being an 'Army of One.' True resilience is about how we create interdependence and draw from the strength of those in our tribe."

—DOC SHAUNA SPRINGER, Ph.D., Bestselling Author

"*Arsenal of Hope* is an essential read for anyone trying to understand the effects of PTSD, those struggling to support someone in the depths of their struggle, or those who simply need to know they are not alone."

—KALEA LEHMAN, the Executive Director and Founder,
Military Special Operations Family Collaborative

"I'd like to encourage *anyone* who is living their life affected by PTSD to check it out—it isn't a combat family exclusive reality. Trauma is trauma."

—SARAH KELLY, Special Operations
Warrior Family Advocate

"PTS is a soldier's invisible enemy because it's an internal response to the emotional, mental, and physical realities of battles...the material in *Arsenal of Hope* has solutions that benefit the entire family. They deserve all we can do to help."

—TONY LA RUSSA, Hall of Fame Manager,
Three-Time World Series Champion

"Jen Satterly shares compelling and powerful personal stories on the insidious nature of post-traumatic stress...she shines a bright and unwavering light on the path to recovery, forgiveness, and freedom."

—COLONEL STU FARRIS, American
Soldier, Husband, and Father

CONTENTS

AUTHOR'S NOTE

COVID-19 HAS SUNK ITS FANGS INTO *MILLIONS* OF PEOPLE, MANY of whom are now enduring extreme levels of trauma and the ensuing biological response known as post-traumatic stress disorder. While this book is written through the lens of Jennifer Satterly's experiences, largely built on her life with the military's Special Forces, the content is intended for anyone suffering from PTSD, no matter the source. The final chapter specifically addresses how social upheaval, including the pandemic and the race riots, is creating or amplifying PTSD in multiple populations.

But it is important to note that our soldiers and veterans and their families have been struggling with this crushing syndrome on a large scale for centuries. Between eleven and twenty out of every one hundred veterans who have seen conflict are now believed to have complex post-traumatic stress disorder, according to the US Department of Veterans Affairs. This means roughly 20 percent of our military families are suffering, because these soldiers don't suffer alone. PTSD brings everybody in the house chaos and pain. The more severe the veteran's symptoms, the more distress and violence found in the home. In September 2019, the

Pentagon released the first-ever report on military spouse and child suicides; the Department of Defense 2018 Annual Suicide Report revealed that 123 spouses and sixty-three children took their own lives in 2017.

Those numbers are alarming and sickening, but there are (conservatively) *half a million* families who are living with a wounded warrior and the nightmare of PTSD, military children and spouses facing prolonged abuse or even violence from a loved one (based on a 2014 Rand Corp. study of PTSD in Iraq/Afghanistan vets). War is not left in the sand overseas—it attaches itself to the soldier, an oftentimes-invisible parasite, and settles into our homes, where our men, women, and children are suffering largely in silence.

Family members must start advocating for themselves. There is help out there, but you have to ask for it, and you have to work for it. You deserve a safe roof over your head just as much as your soldier does.

FOREWORD

THERE ARE A FEW RULES I'VE LIVED BY MOST OF MY ADULT LIFE. One I hold sacred is to protect the secrecy of my unit and what we went through together, so when my wife first suggested I write a book, I refused. Then Jen finally convinced me that saving the lives of others stuck in the hellish depths of PTSD, like I had been, was worth more than the fear of judgment. Putting things down on paper wasn't easy, especially the darkest times, but those who read *All Secure* quickly discovered that the real hero of my story was Jen. Not only did she save my life, walking with me through my personal hell, but also countless other men and women. Her dedication and determination to help others heal is unmatched. Her story is as powerful as any hero's I know.

Arsenal of Hope is without question just as important as *All Secure*, if not more so. It is eye opening and painful, highlighting the oft-hidden trauma military and veteran spouses endure. The support system provided by those at home is critical not only to soldiers but to this country, and yet is overlooked or ignored. Their burden and stress are tremendous, with no consistent help performing the daily routine of balancing jobs with carting kids off to school or track meets, while also providing love and discipline—and living as a single parent with the constant worry their spouse will not return from overseas.

But the trauma and stress can then triple-fold when the soldier returns, changed and sometimes scary. There are thousands and thousands of families who need our help dealing with the monster that is PTSD.

I have never been prouder of my wife, and that's saying something. This book needs to be in the hands of everyone, military service members, spouses, and family members, but also anyone who suffers from post-traumatic stress.

Jen, my angel, taught me to choose my path and how to be aware and responsible for my response to the world around me. She can help you, too, if you so choose.

—*Tom Satterly*
Retired Command
Sgt. Major Delta Force

INTRODUCTION

Whiskey Tango Foxtrot (Seriously, WTF): How I Became an Unwitting Authority On PTSD

I THOUGHT LOVE HAD TO HURT FOR IT TO BE REAL.

It was...oh hell, it was programmed into me. Childhood trauma and a rough turn in my twenties validated what I thought to be true, that I was unworthy of being loved. Unbeknownst to me, this self-loathing was a core symptom of post-traumatic stress, one that easily takes root and is hard as hell to dig out.

As a young kid, my insecurity was a bullhorn, constantly shouting at me: "Make yourself unseen! Unheard! Make yourself small! Invisible people can't get hurt."

After years of that type of response in the face of the slightest hint of conflict—which didn't do anything except attract bullies in school—I knew I had to change my behavior. As the taunting and harassment only increased, I decided instead of trying to make myself small, I would make myself big. The clown. The attention-seeking, funny wild-child with a false bravado, desperate to be seen and loved. And, of course, that led me into whole slew of trouble.

Finally, I shouted back at my insecurity: "I will not be a victim, dammit!"

And, for good or bad, that became my mantra.

I am grateful for those experiences in my early years. Don't get me wrong, I definitely was not grateful when I was in an abusive or downright traumatic situation. However, the bad stuff I went through prepared me for the greatest love of my life, and then how to help save that love. While embedded with Special Operations units, filming large-scale and dangerous Realistic Military Training exercises surrounded by aggressive tough guys, I fell in love with one of them: Command Sergeant Tom Satterly, a senior non-commissioned officer in the most secretive and elite Special Operations unit in the US military. A legend even among other Tier One special operators. Picture a mixture of Jason Bourne, James Bond, and Rambo. In other words, a highly trained, highly deadly soldier. A badass.

Tom and I are the reverse of most couples: we started out in a bad place. It's a miracle we made it at all. The morning after our wedding—married for literally only a few hours—I woke up and told him I wanted him to rip up the marriage certificate and throw it away. I was going home. Alone. The nightmare that had been our wedding night was the final straw. Thankfully, my love and respect for Tom stopped me from leaving that room.

Over the course of twenty years and thousands of missions, he'd rescued hostages; killed and captured high-value targets, including terrorist leaders; and seen his brothers maimed and killed around him while protecting America. I mean, my God, his first combat mission was the Battle of Mogadishu, Somalia (the movie *Black Hawk Down* was based on this battle). Despite the infinite respect due to this wounded warrior, however, no one would blame me for walking away. Our love story could have been over.

I don't give up easily. I'm stubborn and dig in when faced with a challenge. So, I drew my line in the sand and, luckily, Tom stepped up to it and negotiated, saving our relationship. We decided to put in the work to preserve what we knew was real and important, and then we did that long, hard work. Awareness of what you have and what is worth fighting for is one thing, and an important thing, but it's an entirely different thing to roll up your sleeves and get to work through the hard stuff. Today, we're like newlyweds or best friends who fell in love. We are not without our challenges, but we are nowhere near where we began. With me, most everything is backward or mismatched, so this isn't as surprising to me as it is to others.

I always took on the broken and wounded as my own. In fact, I joke with Tom that when we met, my PTSD was attracted to his PTSD. Hurt is attracted to hurt. It's familiar. Oddly comfortable. Many of the veteran spouses I work with or know also come from troubled childhoods or pasts.

I think in part because I couldn't save myself when I was young, I found others that needed saving. Or maybe it was because I didn't want to or wasn't ready to do the work on myself. A distraction. Since I was a kid, I'd obsessed over proving myself to others. The relentless bullying and abuse, the learning disabilities I didn't know I had, the freckles that I was told to cover in order to be pretty, and so on…I needed to know I was worthy, that I was good enough. I struggled to shake that yoke; it was so much easier to help others. When I helped someone and they felt better, I felt better. Like I could actually do something right. It became my drug of choice.

When it came to fixing me, I didn't know where to start. Years of talk therapy in high school had helped but didn't provide me the road map of where I needed to go to really transform my pain. I'd released some of the poison, but then I was left with empty places that I had no idea how to fill. I stopped trying to heal myself. Yet, with Tom, all I did was try. And try and try. Other than being a mother, I've never tried at anything harder and with more conviction than I did for Tom. For us.

In the end, I realized every step I took for Tom ended up helping me, as well.

He's a warrior. But only recently did I own that I, too, am a warrior. We both fight for that which we love. Because of that, we both have scars. We both have armor. These battles prepared me for Tom and for the others I love in my tribe, my unlikely family, those who push and take risks and fight for something bigger than themselves.

That's how, against all odds, I ended up working in Special Operations training missions.

While combat camera was used overseas and sometimes in training exercises, it was by no means common place to have a camera around Special Operations units. Their large-scale Realistic Military Training exercises were classified, critical, and dangerous. I filmed every single moment from the time the unit landed at the airfield, set up their JOC (joint operations center), meetings, intel, planning missions, and training, and then flowed along when they would shoot the enemies or save hostages or bust drug cartels. I came prepared for days in the field, dressed in Crye MultiCam pants, trekking boots, and a staff t-shirt, silently shadowing the warriors' every move over rough or dangerous terrain.

I was a fly on the wall. I never flirted or drew attention to myself; to be anything less than a professional jeopardized the exercise. I was sensitive to being the only female most of the time. I wanted them to see me as a quiet expert they could trust, not just "that blonde girl with a camera." I came home with burn marks from hot metal, a black eye once or twice, a sprained ankle from falling down a hill after being accidentally knocked down by two team members—I shoved down the pain, brushed off my pants, and followed them. They didn't know and I didn't say a word. They were going to have to face much worse than that. They'd been through worse. I did not bitch about my minor wounds or hurts, not even the accidental gun butt to my face. I motioned for the guys to go on, no worries, and they kept going. So did I. I took my job seriously. The footage was used to evaluate their tactics and techniques. This would help them get better. This would help keep them alive.

Still, I found myself a stranger in a strange land. I never thought in a million years I would work alongside the military.

I was a creative type. I'd worked in the male-dominated advertising world all my life, but the men there were also creatives, mostly even-tempered and laid-back. Straight out of college, I became the only female art director at a highly competitive, testosterone-filled design agency with wannabe soldiers (an obscene amount of war movies and video games were played at work, and a gold-plated Uzi hung on the wall). I could only take that kind of senseless bullshit for so long. I built my client base and not so quietly left to start up my own boutique advertising and film/photography studio. I wanted to have the freedom to work with the clients I wanted to work with, and I no longer wanted to put up with the bullying behavior that had become relentless toward several of the younger staff. I decided to be the first to go, middle finger up as I left. No more abuse for me, fuck you very much.

I approached the military with the idea of filming their large-scale Realistic Military Training exercises. The idea was met with a lot of raised eyebrows, but I'd worked in sports marketing and knew that players and coaches reviewed games constantly, in order to learn from their mistakes. I believed that embedding with Navy Seals, Green Berets, and Army Rangers as they ran through dangerous, crucial combat and rescue scenarios would provide birds-eye footage that would provide life-saving information. So, after years of advertising in the commercial sector, I helped form an elite Special Operations military contracting company and became Director of Film and Photography.

Yet, though I knew I was doing important work, I didn't go into it with the respect for the soldiers the way I should have. I judged. But that didn't last for long.

This was life or death. All the time, that weight was there. The exercises had to be as realistic as possible, so, while training to rescue others, people died. The first exercise I went on had to be shut down on day one when a SEAL was killed in a vehicle accident. The Mine-Resistant Ambush Protected vehicle (an MRAP, an armored tank-like car) rolled and he was killed. Another two were killed in a helicopter crash. It didn't escape me that I could be hurt, badly, during these weeks with the boys (there weren't a lot of women in Special Operations combat roles).

Mostly what I saw working with the Special Operations units was a high level of quiet and even-toned professionalism. Though I was chewed out more than once by mid-level command for being there—filming wasn't common practice, and the leadership didn't always tell the guys on the ground about me—I never really saw people yell. When I did, it stood out, like the time a former unit member ripped into a staff member in charge of the veterans who were there to role-play. The woman got lippy one too many times. I was wide-eyed, as was everyone on the film crew. The Special Op soldier got in her face and screamed a long string of insults, his face red and his breathing fast. It was an oh-shit moment. What was this guy going to do? It became clear to me…these men might be professional soldiers, but they can also be loose cannons. This guy had been through a lot of combat missions, for a long time.

His reaction, I came to find out, was typical for combat trauma left untreated.

That kind of break in a professional military setting isn't common at all. There is a formality in the military: ranks and orders and a way things are done. It has to be respected and followed. People could die if not. Most of what I saw was a high level of attention to detail and professionalism. A respect for each other, even when they disagreed. After the mission, they would do very detailed and direct AAR (after action reviews), not holding back punches about what someone did wrong. In fact, you never heard what anyone did right—doing their job right wasn't something to be rewarded, it was expected. They'd have it out, cuss and yell, and then get right back to business.

The expectations for physical and mental acuity were high, and they were met. The soldiers were almost cold, emotionless. Matter-of-fact. This was a black-and-white world, a place where emotional decisions could get people killed. Humans make emotional decisions and have emotional reactions to situations; soldiers are intensely trained to deny access to any emotion. There was little place for it—except anger. Anger seemed to be an emotion that was normal, though that always made me uncomfortable. When things went a little out of control on a training mission, anger was an appropriate response. Then back to normal. I never wanted to see anyone upset or angry, especially with me. I stayed out of the way.

When I started working alongside Special Operations, it was thrilling. The veil of secrecy had lifted, I was seeing what very few civilians would see. I took the responsibility seriously. I would get annoyed when other moms would tease, "Oooh, going out with the Navy Seals again, huh? I bet you see some serious hotties!" But it was not like that. I was not going to look at abs. I saw young men, some who looked so young at the start and then seemed to age over the course of the job. I saw seriousness. I saw intense concentration. I saw professionalism. This was not the beach volleyball scene out of *Top Gun*, this was life-or-death training.

Nothing annoyed me more than when role-players tried to act like one of the guys on the teams. I never tried to be like the soldiers, to act like them, use their lingo, or try to get in on their inside jokes. They were a tribe who earned their tabs the hard way. Why would I try to act like I was their equal when it came to combat? I'd never seen, smelled, or tasted combat. I'd never heard the crack and snap of a live bullet nearly hit my head, over and over again. I never saw a friend beg for his life and then for his mother as he bled out. Over and over again, these soldiers had endured combat and danger and a level of stress I had never experienced. I never knew the longing of home for months at a time, and then the longing to go back into battle. I never knew any of what it took to survive urban warfare or jungle warfare or any warfare, and I thought it disrespectful to pretend like someone who had.

Realistic Military Training consisted of sixteen-hour days, seven days a week. It was hot and sweaty and bug filled. We went to places like abandoned warehouses, dilapidated hospitals and institutions, mansions destroyed by hurricanes, old jails, and deserted islands.

After an assault on a target was complete, we would drag ourselves to a hotel, take a quick shower to get off the filth from the warehouse and bug spray and dirt and sweat, sleep for three or four hours, and get back up. Take another shower to wake up. Get packed. Meet up with the group of role-players and contractors to review the day's list of to-dos and what was needed for that night's hit, then head out in a convoy to the next town. Set up the target, usually in a dirty place no one would mind if the doors were blown out, the windows smashed, or a bunch of noise was made by gunfire and helos.

No one sat around. If they did, they didn't last long. There's constant movement during setup and everyone is involved. Role-player females get dressed in local garb and help set up rooms, like a fake cocaine packing room in which the women would be dressed in nude suits, making bricks of coke out of baking powder, cling wrap, and duct tape. Or in an Afghan village setting, where they might be hanging sheets in windows, setting up a fire pit and cooking local foods and drink, speaking only in their national language. The Opposing Force (OPFOR) would get to work, loading and cleaning weapons, then dress in their terrorist or militia or drug cartel clothes. The Pyro Techniques team (PYRO) would be making and setting trip wires or putting suicide vests on the bad-guy role-player (vests that would simulate exploding with a loud bang and shooting out raw meat and fake blood).

The Target Controller would be making sure everything was getting done that needed to get done, including helping set up the Opposing Force strategies and talking to our company guys back in the joint operations center. A JOC is where they would plan the nightly missions and watch the intelligence surveillance reconnaissance (ISR) supplied by drones flying overhead, showing the action at the target. The Target Controller would get a call, text, or radio traffic: have the OPFOR start pulling security, have the women move around the village, and so on. From the time the target was prepped and set and the mission began, there was no break in role-playing, even though it could be several hours before the SEALs or Green Berets would show up to take down the target. Those hours could be tedious. Sitting and waiting for dark, for the mission to begin. But begin it would, and the stress didn't alleviate until it was over.

One July mission, we traveled from Savannah to Jacksonville and (no surprise) it was hot, humid, and we were covered in bugs. That night, the FBI joined the mission training, trying to disarm a chemical weapon. We were in an abandoned machine shop with a fuel tank from the space shuttle sitting on the property. It was massive and pretty cool to see up close.

I loved having the chance to explore these places: abandoned buildings, historical sites, and haunted houses, but especially old hospitals or old schools with books and papers and things left behind. I would often photograph the oddities I'd find, like a dentist chair with the medical equipment still sitting out, as if someone just got up and left during a filling and no one cleaned it up for forty years. Or a school room with papers still in the desks from the 1960s, reminding me of the footage I'd seen from Chernobyl. The small bits of history fascinated me.

At one point that night in July, I was pulled out to film the disarming of the weapon of mass destruction. I set my camera up opposite the FBI agent hunched over the weapon.

"Fucking motherfucking fuck. Can someone fucking get the light over here so I can fucking see fucking better or get a-fucking-nother one. Fuck. I need my fucking laptop, fucking sitting right fucking here, not there. Fucking move."

It was intense. He was being filmed while under extreme pressure to perform; it was a bad scenario for him. "I don't fucking care who you fucking actually are and who the fuck you fucking work for, get the fuck out of my area and get that fucking camera out of here right fucking now."

With that, I walked away. He was spinning out. I would usually politely and professionally push back when challenged, since I was part of the contract and the command expected to see footage. I was never a bitch about it, but I'd get that footage. It was my job. However, I knew this was not the time to push. He saw me as chaos, an entity outside the scope of his control, and it triggered his PTSD.

So many of the men and women coming through training were dealing with PTSD. If a breakdown happened, it was like a train about to bust off the rails—you don't want to be anywhere near that kind of collateral damage. I'd witnessed the trauma working at many different levels in these service members, many of whom had become friends.

After I'd been working in Special Operations for almost three years, and I'd come to see the extent of the suffering, I decided I wanted to do something beyond photographing and filming. I wanted to help these warriors. I'd seen firsthand how they were laying their lives on the line and paying for it with immense physical, emotional, and spiritual pain.

I was with Tom by this point. He was now retired, returning as a Tier One Special Operations veteran running the massive training exercises. And we were immersed in his battle with PTSD.

I wasn't a doctor or a therapist, but quite a few of the guys had started talking to me about the treatments that Tom was undergoing and how they were working, and I found the conversations were really helping some of them. The battle was hard, there was no downplaying that.

Tom was working toward healing, one day at a time. He was in a much better and much different place than rock bottom, which is where he'd been when I met him. Anger management therapy was the first big step he'd taken in managing his demons. Then there was addressing the way his body, mind, and spirit were completely wrecked by war.

No one wanted to admit to damage to the mind or spirit, but it *was* easy for him to talk about the physical side—they all did that. It wasn't just the older contractors like Tom who talked about their aches and pains, it was also the young men, already suffering from similar chronic pain. For them, the pain was all-consuming. That's a huge part of the mental game, to deal and cope with chronic, relentless pain that they know will only get worse with time, and the fear of being rendered useless to others because of that pain. That there is little to be done about it is a big part of their mental stress.

A friend I met in a health and wellness Facebook group recently lost her brother. He killed himself after walking out of a VA appointment. The chronic pain after twenty-six years in the Air Force wasn't just depressing, it was devastating to every aspect of his life. He was told by a VA doctor, "There's nothing left we can do for your pain." He went to his car, called his mom, and shot himself. He was a warrior, used to taking care of the problem, and he'd come to believe he was the problem.

I came to see my purpose was not filming RMTs. I'd been in that job, that place, for a purpose, but now it was time to transfer my knowledge and skillset to a new arena, to helping these warriors. But exactly how could I give back?

I loved talking to the guys. "You should try this treatment, read this book, take these supplements your brain needs."

Later, I would get a call: "Hey, it's Matt from Seal Team X. I am having some issues." We would talk for hours, and then, most of the time, I would be asked, "Can you talk to my wife? She doesn't understand, maybe you can help her."

I would always tell them, "I'm not a therapist, I'm not a doctor, but this is my experience with Tom, and this is what we went through and this is what we're doing..." And then I'd take the next call. And the next. I'd show up to the next round of training exercises and would find myself tucked away in a corner talking to a contractor, someone Tom worked with, or a role-player who'd been in Special Operations and was now playing FID force (Foreign Internal Defense, teaching foreign people how to defend themselves) or playing OPFOR (Opposing Forces, or the bad guys). These roles were largely played by trained Special Operations guys and gals. This wasn't the place for amateurs. Not only was I working with active duty Spec Ops, I was working alongside veterans who knew and worked with Tom. They saw a change in him and would ask what he was doing, how was he getting relief.

We'd talk, then it would get deeper. The conversation would shift from treatment discussion to the dark stuff they'd tried to bury. The stories would make me cry. Sometimes they would cry, too.

I'd hear them growl through their tears, "What the *fuuuuuuck*."

I'd say, "No, no, Tom cries, too. For fuck's sake, you're talking about serious pain, pain from loss of friends you loved, pain in your body, pain in your spirit, your mind. Tell your story. Let it out. It's poison."

Someone would mention an issue to Tom, and he'd say, "Go talk to Jen." I loved it, I felt like I was making a difference to people who deserved the help. All of my self-taught research, time with these warriors, and PTSD treatments in our home could go so much further. I was useful in a way I'd never felt useful before. This was the focus I wanted to take now.

I also desperately wanted to be home more with my kids, and so I came up with a plan. I became a certified health coach, to better understand the role nutrition plays in physical and mental health, and Tom and I co-founded the All Secure Foundation, donating our money, time, and efforts to serve the Special Operations warriors and their families, as well as help them heal from the invisible wounds from combat.

Over time, and with endless practice, we have developed an arsenal of tricks and tactics for taking on PTSD, side by side. Here is what I have learned.

ONE

It's Not You, It's You: The Biology of PTSD

THE OTHER DAY, TOM CAME ACROSS AN OLD POCKETKNIFE, staring at it as he flipped it open and shut.

"You okay?" I asked.

"Yeah. It's just that I had to use this on a bomb maker once." He paused. "He's not doing that anymore."

My stomach dropped. I had to consciously remind myself that without retired Delta Force Command Sgt. Major Tom Satterly and his actions, many more would have died. It's not fair for me to bring my perspective to bear on Tom's experiences, not when he has dealt with the worst of humanity, men who stoned their wives to death, threw acid in the face of a child, or blew up markets full of innocent people. I have no place in his stories. I cannot think, "I don't know if I could have cut a man." Instead, my place is here, beside him, giving him a safe place to release the ugliness. I don't have to empathize, just be present, non-judgmental.

He flipped the knife shut and swung around to face me. "Bad guys like him need to die; I don't feel bad, you know."

Because I love Tom Satterly, with a love that is unimaginably big and beautiful, and I want this man to be my partner for the rest of my life, I had to learn to embrace Tom for exactly who he is, not who I thought he should be. It's not my place to make him see his experiences from another perspective. Tom *does* understand the human condition, he can love his fellow man, but he has to be able to make snap judgments on who is good and who is a killer and neutralize that threat without hesitation. He, and soldiers like him, take out the bomb makers, the men with machine guns spraying down crowds, the men who tortured his teammates. Should he feel bad about neutralizing that type of threat, once and for all? Let the moral injuries wreak havoc on his ability to function? No. Without him and his ability to live with that decision, our country would not be safe, and the world would be far less secure.

The challenge of my relationship with Tom has opened a part of me I didn't know existed: the ability to love Tom for who he is. And the ability to love myself for who I am. As we were and as we are today.

Also, I definitely had to let go of pre-conceived notions about the military. Despite the fact that I ended up working with Special Ops people and then married to Tom, I grew up in a house that was academic-oriented and viewed guns as abhorrent. Though my dad and brother were Air Force, my mother nurtured in us the belief that military guys were uneducated rednecks who loved chasing women, drinking excessively, and had a thirst for violence. They were into partying and routine infidelity. In fact, I made a rule when I was young to never marry a rock star, a pro athlete, or a military man, all of whom seemed like more trouble than they were worth.

Sure, some soldiers can be assholes, they can be mean…but, if they are this way, it's because of what is necessary to get the job done. They are this way for us. And we aren't actively helping them assimilate or find mental clarity when they get home. My experience with Special Operations taught me to bring compassion instead of judgment, to admire and respect the hell out of Tom and his tribe, now part of my own tribe.

I don't judge him. Well, okay, that's not true. I'm human, and humans judge. I can say honestly, though, that I try fervently not to bring judgment to his story or his decisions, and he tries to do the same with me. We often fail, but we are getting better with awareness and with practice. I want to help him lead the best life he can, the life he deserves. After all, he's thrown himself into a volley of bullets hundreds of times for this country and, in doing so, he has sacrificed not just his well-being on the field, but also his sense of safety and place and well-being in his own house. He sacrificed not only Christmas mornings with his children, he's given up his peace of mind, something most of us can't fathom.

After twenty-five years of combat service, he is retired, but the war followed him home.

I was forced to deal with that truth when Tom and I hit rock bottom in our relationship. The man I loved had complex post-traumatic stress. I was shocked to discover that, after finally acknowledging the nature of PTSD, it was evident that

I, too, suffered from PTSD, thanks to childhood abuse and a rape that I had suppressed—and that, while living with the symptoms of Tom's trauma, I had developed secondary complex post-traumatic stress.

Never one to back down in face of a challenge, the anthropologist and researcher in me jumped on the science behind the disorder, getting to know the biology of the condition. And the counselor in me got busy with self-analysis, so as to better understand Tom and myself. In coming to understand the condition and its consequences, I was able to move forward. Hopefully, you can begin to do the same.

Of course, I wasn't thinking of any of this when I first met my husband.

I Should've Known

When I met Tom, signs of his PTSD weren't obvious—but, then again, I hadn't gotten close to him yet.

He was funny and charming. When he told a story, others gathered around, everyone laughing and joining in. He was kind to strangers and friends alike, willing to give them the shirt off his back. Or to take a bullet for them.

He cared for his military family. I loved that he was from this totally different world with a completely different point of view. I loved hearing the stories of the crazy things he had done: hostage rescues, assassinations, terrorist takedowns. He was instrumental in the capture of Saddam Hussein and other high-level terrorist leaders. His past was like the plot of a real-life movie. Action and adventure and cool-guy stuff. I didn't watch military movies, which were too real, too horrific for me, but I enjoyed spy stories, especially the Bond or Bourne movies. Now, here I was, spending time with a real Jason Bourne. It was surreal.

I hadn't seen *Black Hawk Down* when we first met. I remember sitting in my living room with a box of tissues, staring at the images on the screen. Tom's role in that eighteen-hour firefight on the streets of Mogadishu was actually represented by a conglomeration of several actors, who had to portray the active duty Delta Force characters as Rangers, keeping their true identities secret. Watching the reenactment of that hellish battle, the longest sustained firefight since Vietnam, I went through half a box of Kleenex, thinking, "How does anyone come back home okay after that?!"

Well, the short answer is, he didn't come home okay.

When Tom and I first started spending time together, I noticed he drank. A lot. Drinking was his medication, and he never missed a dose. He didn't drink some, he drank it all. Seven days a week. Sometimes he would text me mid-afternoon or at lunch and I could tell he'd already started drinking. Of course, he always denied it.

Like so many of the military spouses, I noticed a change in his personality after drink three, but there was no stopping him. He and the other soldiers drank quickly. I remember a friend of his would order two at a time, like he was afraid they'd run out of beer or that someone was going to steal his drink before he had a chance to gulp it down. I always thought Tom drank to numb the pain, but he drank, we both drank, to actually *feel* something, to feel happy, feel alive. He wanted the alcohol to make him weightless, to take him anywhere other than where he was, yet he could never quite get drunk enough to get away from himself, at least not for long.

Then we started falling for each other, romance creeping in. I wasn't used to the way he doted on me, with constant attention, affection, and complements. He texted me obsessively, and I thought it charming to be wanted and needed for a change, not as a creative partner or a parent, but as a woman who desperately wanted to be seen. After a short while, however, the reins of his attention started to tighten. If I didn't answer right away or he didn't like my response, Tom would snap back with a remark that wasn't appropriate. I would confront him, but he'd defend it, claiming it was my fault, that I'd done something to deserve the anger and rudeness. Sometimes he was downright cruel.

I questioned myself nonstop: Am I doing the right thing by dating this guy? Will he stop being mean and controlling? Will he lay off the booze? Will he start taking care of himself? Will he hurt me? Is he safe? Why am I with someone who talks to me this way? Why am I back with an angry person?

We were trapped in a cycle. Apologies, sincere and honest, full of regret and shame. He was like a puppy that got caught chewing a shoe and was popped in the nose with a newspaper. He'd offer up big eyes and a promise that he wouldn't do it again. "I'm sorry" was just as common as "I love you." I heard both several times a day.

But the girl who liked to help those in trouble, those hurting, was a big part of me, it always had been. A therapist once told me that I chose Tom because I had never dealt with my childhood trauma. It sounded a bit basic, the girl who was abused ending up with an abusive man. I never like being basic.

Our connection was undeniable. It was intense and sincere. We would go on long walks, holding hands and talking about our future; we would go out and play darts and dance to slow songs closer than I'd thought humanly possible; and he would even dance with me during the fast songs, laughing and moving on the floor with kids half our age. He made me laugh like no one ever has, with that deep belly kind of laugh. He constantly complimented me, told me (and continues to tell me every morning), "Good morning, beautiful, I'm so lucky to have you." Our sex life was off the charts. Both of us talked about how we felt transported while we made love, a deep kind of connection neither of us had ever felt with anyone else, a cosmic connection beyond ourselves. Beyond this world.

There is so much good here, so much great here, that I never want to be without that kind of love. I never want to be without him. Except when I do.

When we first met, I wanted him to will away the behavior. I'd yell, "Just stop doing this! Get over it. You have to move on, and you have to do it now!"

I'd think, *Change now. Be kind, don't yell, don't insult, don't get so angry, be patient, don't sweat the fucking small stuff.* My relentless pushing him to change only confirmed what he already believed: *I'm not good enough as I am.*

I didn't know this at the time. I truly was coming from a place of desperation, trying to save him and our relationship. *I will change him so he won't want to hurt me, to hurt himself. I will love him enough for the both of us. I will rescue him. I will save him.*

This made him feel weak, unable to understand why he couldn't change, why his willpower was so lacking that he couldn't just stop. This enraged him. This hurt him. It shamed and embarrassed him. He wanted to be a different man, he wanted to be the man I deserved. He told me daily. He hated that he couldn't reign in his destructive behavior at home when he could maintain absolute control on a battlefield.

Tom buried his despair in more alcohol, in accepting and returning the attention he received from women, anything that made him feel alive, feel happy, even just for a moment or a night. The reckless behavior wasn't to numb anything; he already felt numb. He drank or flirted or smoked or drove like a madman to feel alive, to feel anything.

It was then that I started to look into PTSD and the biology of it. As I worked alongside hundreds of warriors who were exhibiting the exact same symptoms and behaviors—and, I mean, story after story was nearly identical—I realized this was much more complicated than simply having the willpower to change. Something was happening biologically to make Tom this way, something deep and not understood by us.

What PTSD Looks Like

Let me first show you what it looks like on a small, daily basis, this PTSD playing out in households across the US. The individual straws that build up to eventually break the camel's back.

When my husband and I were first together, neither of us realized the extent that Tom, a twenty-five-year combat veteran, was battling with full-blown complex post-traumatic stress. And I definitely did not understand that complex secondary post-traumatic stress disorder was messing with my ability to be a good partner. Who knew that was even a thing? Our early days together were not always pretty. I often used to think, *This relationship is absolutely crazy, toxic, and if anyone saw what was happening behind these doors, they would find me weak, co-dependent, a victim.* God, I didn't want to be a victim, perceived or real, anymore in my life. And what would people think of him? A terror in his own home, a reckless wrecker of everything that surrounded him. A monster.

In those years, I wanted to be angry with him. I liked it better than feeling afraid of him, of making myself small, like I had when I was a child.

It wasn't rare for a calm and peaceful, even joyful, moment to come crashing down unexpectedly and often unprovoked. For instance, one night we spent quality time snuggled up on the couch comfortably chilling in front of Netflix, until he got up, walked into the kitchen, and shouted, "Why in the *fuck* can't you pick up after yourself?!" As he rinsed the single mug I had left in the sink, he talked to himself, a string of insults flying easily out of his mouth, aimed at me. One after the other, each louder and more agitated, until he was absolutely sure his verbal swings had knocked me down.

This type of random, misplaced rage came out of nowhere. And it happened all the time.

I wanted for him to feel the weight of the baseless words, the flutter of fear he inspired—his training and muscle memory for violent action wasn't lost on me. I needed him to understand it was beyond devastating. Whenever he was insulting me or doing something that was just wrong and maybe wasn't going to stop, I needed him to feel the impossible weight of his words, crushing me like giant boulders I couldn't crawl out from under. I wanted to hold him accountable, and not just until he apologized. I wanted to make sure he understood that it hurt, that it broke me every time. I never knew my heart could break so many times and still continue to beat.

It wasn't okay, hitting below the belt like he did. Pulling out all the stops, not quitting until his mission to regain control was successful. In order to do so, he hurt me in ways that only the closest person in the world could. And for what? A dish left in the sink, a sock on the living room floor, a change of plans last minute.

Why in the hell was I being called terrible names? If the bed wasn't made quickly enough, there were a string of insults about my looks, or my beliefs, or my past. Why? He deserved all of the respect in the world for what he had done for this country, the danger he had faced...but didn't I deserve just a little respect myself, as a goddamn human being?

Was it really worth the fight?

In response to that question, my thoughts would go round and round.

I would have conversations like the following with myself—often out loud, but under my breath:

> I'll beat it into his head, if I have to. I have to be strong and hold my ground. He has to feel ashamed to understand that he's fucked up. Again. He went too far. Again. I hate when his eyes narrow at me, cold and scary. I've told him a thousand times, why can't he stop approaching

me with so much anger? Why can't he just stop or, better yet, just not start in the first place?

Fine, I'll play. I will do what it takes to make him ashamed. I'll give the cold shoulder or maybe I'll bring up things he did to me in the past to validate my anger.

I will yell at him: See, you do this all the time, like this one time or that one time.

Now I'll bring up some friends to prove I'm right: Even Jack said you're an ass, the guys you worked with agree.

What good is this? Now he's mad. Like, really mad. His veins pop out of his forehead and he goes a dark red. His hands clench, and I know he wants to hit me. Sometimes he punches the wall next to my face or slams the table to release the energy. Bang.

I can cry and get small like a mouse. I oftentimes do. Not say another goddamn word, certainly stop firing back. I can sink into my chair or try to leave the room. But he won't be happy with that. He's the pursuer, and I am the withdrawer. Small makes him feel bigger. Quiet makes him louder.

Mousey behavior is disgusting to him. Weak. Something to crush.

So, I can get bigger. I can get physical, too. He comes near me again and I'm going to fucking slap his face. I'll hit first. Maybe that will wake him up. Maybe that will earn me some respect, to know I am not a target to mess with.

But all it does is confirm in his mind that I actually am a target.

Now we're in a tussle. Like a real fight, grabbing, pulling, pushing each other. Enraged. So much of my pent-up anger explodes. Wrath, that is all I feel. I don't even care if he hurts me at this point. If he grabs me, I kick him. This is a very dangerous game to play with someone who can kill me in a single move, someone who in a fit of rage is capable of great acts of violence; others in his unit have killed their wives under similar situations. This is never far from my mind. Even as I physically fight back, at my lowest, I don't care if I die. I am broken now, just like him.

Then, a breath. Just one pause. And then the release is over and the tears start. The immediate flood of guilt, shame, embarrassment. He says he'll leave me. That he won't put me through this again. That he is a monster. That he doesn't deserve to live.

Both of us in tears, now I'm grabbing him to stay: Dear God, don't walk out the door!

If he leaves now, he'll drive like a madman into a tree. He'll shoot himself. Keep him here. Hide his guns.

Pleading and begging through the pain: I'm okay. We're okay. I swear I'm fine.

And then Tom would come back. My Tom. His face muscles would relax. Behind a sheen of tears, the black in his eyes morphed back to blue. Tom would return and Crawler (Tom's call sign) would evaporate.

Crawler is a fucking asshole at all times, always intense. Tom becomes this someone else in order to do the work he has to do: killing, capturing, interrogating. That man doesn't belong in a house, he belongs to the war. He's frightening. He is the warrior and, with the flip of a switch, I would become the enemy, to be destroyed.

Can Tom control the flip of the switch? If he can, does he know how? Or maybe he doesn't want to? That last was the worst thought of all.

I perpetually walked on eggshells. Or, more aptly, I was stepping lightly through a minefield. You can't predict what an unpredictable man will do. It'll make you crazy trying. For years, I tried. I failed. It made me more insecure. More isolated. I kept myself distant from him, to protect myself, but also distant from our friends and family, to protect Tom.

On the day our fight turned into that physical tussle, and then I watched Crawler turn back into my Tom, my husband, I leaned against the wall, shaking, no more fight left in me.

This was over a cup in the sink. Again.

In that moment, I had to decide. Would I keep loving this man? Looking at the face of the wounded warrior before me, I knew I could not live without him. He was my person. So, I decided I would love him, even when I didn't want to. Even if the outside world would never understand why.

But I would not live like this, either. I had grown to love someone else through this: myself. And I wouldn't allow anyone I loved to be treated this way. Neither would Tom. We had to be strong enough to change. Thank God he agreed.

If he had not been willing to put in the work, I wouldn't have continued to do so, not by myself. You can't force someone to get well. You can, however, show them the path and, even better, you can walk beside them. Sometimes leading the way, sometimes following, but the decision has to be made by the individual to put in the work to retrain, to heal: a year of weekly therapy sessions, including emotionally focused therapy as a couple; TMS, transcranial magnetic stimulation, therapy for his depression and anxiety; adapting to a nutritious diet with much-needed supplements for his physical pain, his brain function, and hormonal balance; and finding our purpose, which both of us felt meant giving back. Repeatedly sharing his stories so that he no longer had nightmares or tears when he told them. So much work over time…it was worth it. Things changed in us both.

Stacey Stone, our therapist, told us, "When one of you 'wins,' the relationship loses."

I wrote it down on a Post-it. I put it on our mirror in the bathroom. I journaled about it.

I had to decide if PTSD would win. I was fucking tired of losing to a condition. Years of battles. When would this war be over?

Most likely the trauma of war will always be embedded in his mind. *Okay, so how do I deal with this life we have? How do I thrive? How am I happy? How are we happy? Can I hold out? Can he?*

"When I win, the relationship loses," I muttered to myself. So, I shifted my perception, seeing Tom and I as a unit, a whole thing, something to protect above all else. Protecting it from him, from me, from PTSD. I became the defender and protector of Tom and Jen, something worth fighting for.

I started to see Crawler as someone separate from Tom, the husband and best friend I loved and adored. When he came out, I called him by his name: "Crawler doesn't need to handle the kitchen right now. Either Tom or I will do it."

Sounds a bit batshit crazy, but you have to be a little crazy to fight PTSD. You have to embrace the crazy.

It worked; it stopped the negative cycle. This method isn't a 100 percent cure all, but it helps us. A lot. I never use Crawler as an insult, not if Tom is just being Tom. Ever. I respect Crawler and his service, I just don't want him in my kitchen.

If you are dealing with PTSD in your home, so much of this will look familiar to you.

The Science behind PTSD: Simple, Complex, and Secondary

The following statistics were addressed in the Author's Note but bear repeating: Between eleven and twenty out of every one hundred veterans who have seen conflict are now believed to have complex post-traumatic stress disorder, according to the US Department of Veterans Affairs, which means at least 20 percent of our military families are suffering through chaos and pain, and sometimes violence or threats of suicide, in their homes.

Our soldiers hate the term PTSD, in particular the word "disorder." They don't want to be labeled anything that makes them sound sick, like they can't go back into the field, or weak, like they couldn't kick the enemy's ass when they need to. Because of that, some medical or support agencies are now referring to PTSD as PTS, or as something else entirely, like occupational stress injury. Semantics do matter, I get that, especially in a world where you have to have a strong ego just as much as a strong body, but for the sake of understanding the condition and to help us all get a handle on our wounded warriors, I'm going to stick with the terminology we know for this book. On a side note, though, myself and our non-profit organization, All Secure Foundation, always refer to it as PTS.

Response to trauma differs from one individual to the next. Why? Because. That's why. That's the best I can do. One person can live through their house being destroyed around them by a tornado and be perfectly fine in a few days. Another person living through the same incident may spend the rest of their life triggered by high winds. However, response also depends on whether or not the trauma is a one-time incident or occurs over time.

According to the Volunteers of America, post-traumatic stress disorder may arise when people experience a traumatic event such as death, threatened death, serious injury, medical trauma, or actual or threatened sexual violence. The symptoms involve terror, helplessness, numbness, withdrawal, and confusion, and can be triggered at a later date. When there is a single event that causes the condition, that is referred to as simple PTSD. However, soldiers (and first responders) who are diagnosed with a stress disorder are generally considered to have complex PTSD;

combat vets generally endure repeated, prolonged physical, emotional, and mental trauma. Their symptoms are more severe, often adding depression, substance abuse, infidelity, personality changes, paralysis, difficulty in making decisions, self-hatred, shame spiraling, distrust, fatigue, sleeping and eating disorders, or aggression against self and others.

Our warriors who live with PTSD are dealing with a condition that initiates a limited ability to function as a parent or partner, creating prolonged stress within the family. Secondary PTSD is sometimes referred to as "compassion fatigue," because those caring for traumatized patients can be emotionally and physically pushed past their breaking point. Family members with military PTSD in the household are sometimes diagnosed with secondary complex PTSD, having endured over a long period of time the harmful behaviors that the soldier cannot control.

A family member with SPTSD might do what I did, try to make themselves small or invisible, and then rage when the resentment gets too much. There will be depression and imbalanced sleep habits. I found myself sleeping a lot, depressed and avoiding the conflicts. Then there were the times I couldn't sleep more than a few hours at a time, twisting and turning with anxiety. There will likely be paranoia and a tenseness, now that a personal sense of safety is threatened for long periods, and the knowledge that a verbal or even physical attack can come at any time, leading to hopelessness and deeper isolation. In children, we see them become silent and withdrawn, or they may go the other way and behave aggressively at inappropriate times. These spouses and children devise ways to protect their sense of self, many of which are unhealthy and develop into behavioral patterns. For some, there is self-medicating with alcohol or drugs or overeating. Whatever it takes.

Many of these symptoms and the coping mechanisms are discussed in more detail in later chapters, including a chapter specifically dealing with the consequences to military children and what can be done to help them.

Understand that PTSD is a brain disorder, and it is a *biological* condition. It is similar to brain cancer in that the brain chemistry and processes have been impacted by no fault of the sufferer, and there is no easy, sure-fire cure. A person with a brain tumor is not blamed for the injury to their brain or the resulting symptoms. When a cancer patient's personality changes, we blame the disease and don't expect that the patient can just "snap out of it" without medical intervention. Rightly so. This is also accurate for our soldiers with PTSD. They did not ask for their brain functionality to be altered, nor do they have the ability to just "snap out of it." *Willpower, no matter how strong, cannot resolve the biological issues.* The condition must be treated as a serious condition that can be overcome, but only with persistence and hard work, including re-wiring brain chemistry and ingrained behaviors.

We know that long-term stress has powerful, negative effects on the body. Part of a soldier's complex PTSD is called moral injury, an age-old concept that is finally getting talked about in medical terms. Combat soldiers are often asked to break their own moral code, like when they must hurt or kill an enemy. Hurt or kill another *human*. Though asked to do so for the greater good, these soldiers are left to ponder if they are now themselves evil, if something inside of them is broken, never to be whole again. I remember when one of the guys I was working with said to me, "Well, I'm going to Hell for all the shit I've done, so what does it matter what I do now?" This sense of moral injury kicks off many of the worst of the PTSD symptoms. This crisis of the mind and soul has been happening to soldiers since there were wars, and yet we are just now providing terminology, definitions, and hopefully, healing processes. Healing modalities will be discussed at length later on, but for now, just know there is hope.

When I went to health coaching school, I had lightning-bolt moments. I would scream through the house, "Ohhhhhh my gaaaawwwd, *Tom*, I just learned…" It was so much of a relief to stumble across something that could help him, something that explained why he felt the way he did.

One of the biggest ah-ha moments had to do with reading about his mind and his body and how they were working to protect him. The parasympathetic and sympathetic nervous system, which elicits the fight, flight, or freeze response, was switched on, but it never went off. This meant his brain could not distinguish a perceived threat from an actual threat. Everything, including the overreaction to the cup in the sink, was a biological response to "get safe and secure." In combat, there is nothing but chaos, and the way out of it is to create order. Do you ask a terrorist to politely get on the floor after they just tried to shoot you? Do you calmly ask for a time out when your best friend was dropped by a bullet ten feet in front of you?

The funny thing is, Tom was very collected in combat. Many who served under him said that his calm and confident voice over the radio got them through some of the most horrible scenarios they were involved in. He did well in the chaos of war; he was one of the most well-trained soldiers in one of the most elite units in the world. Everything had a system or a way of moving, it was choreographed like a dance. When things went bad, like they often did, there was no time for screaming and freaking out—you simply responded how you were trained to respond. It was fucking life or death.

But chaos at home, like kids screaming and dogs barking and someone at the door and dinner is burnt...well, there is no playbook for that, there is no training for the randomness of everyday life. There are no buddies with you, your team is not there. You're essentially alone, and the brain immediately reads this as danger and that the threat needs to be controlled or eliminated. Unfortunately, "family" is now the threat and is dealt with in the same manner as any threat overseas: bluntly, coarsely, with piss and vinegar and then anger or violence when the situation doesn't quickly go from chaos to order.

"Why am I so angry all the time?" That is the number one question I am asked by hundreds of combat warriors. "Why do I react this way to stupid shit? God, why can't I get control of my anger?"

I often respond with, "What tools did you need to survive in combat?"

"Anger, violence, aggression, speed of action, and did I mention violence?"

"How did you get home and, more importantly to you no doubt, how did you bring your brothers home?"

"I relied on my training. I acted quickly and violently."

The brain develops muscle memory. If a person repeats the same action over and over again, they will become good at it. Ten thousand repetitions make an expert, some say. A soldier trains, fights, trains, fights. The brain sees the trained actions and behaviors as the new normal. Just like when you knock over a glass and, without thinking, you reach to grab it. When that soldier is back at home and the morning they have planned is interrupted by the kids yelling and then the dog eats their favorite shoe, that soldier's brain responds like it was trained to respond—with anger, aggression, and sometimes violence. It's a natural response not only to trauma but to training.

If your warrior is battling PTSD and your house is under attack, like I said, there is hope. You do have weapons in your arsenal against this thing, you just don't know it yet. I've seen change and real healing, even after some of the worst examples of PTSD tearing apart families.

Right now, you need to know you are not alone, that so many people have gone through this pain with their partners and come out on the other side. This is not a cliché or hyperbole. Believe it. Say it with me: "I am not alone. There is hope."

Here are their stories.

Stories from behind the Thin Green Line

Over the years, I've worked with exceptional people. Daryl is one such person. He is soft-spoken, generous, and funny. He is a deeply spiritual man, even serving as a pastor for a time, and a loving husband and father for over thirty-five years. He is good to those around him, many of whom have no idea how much he has suffered.

He called a few years ago, looking for relief from pain in his joints, but then he opened up about the pain in his soul. He'd served overseas during countless deployments and then at home as a member of an elite SWAT team, observing more than his share of the horrors men do to other men.

One particular combat experience had him in a repeat cycle of nightmares and anxiety. "I can still see the man's face, right up close to me. I can see his blood all over my hands. I can see the white of his eyes. For some reason, I can't get him out of my mind, like the memory is burnt into my brain."

Daryl was talking hand-to-hand combat—something that is actually very rare, much rarer than firefights, and causes far greater mental impact to those who engage in it. Tom talks about this often, how he only had a few hand-to-hand combat fights over the course of his entire career, but it was that being eyeball to eyeball with an enemy who was trying to kill him that bothered him the most. It was so insanely personal.

The more Daryl talked, the more he revealed, and it was absolutely gut-wrenching. So many reasons for him to have PTSD. His son Jonathan, a boy with a big heart, close with his family and friends, had served as a combat medic. He came back from his second deployment a different man, obviously hurting. At twenty-one years of age, he'd seen too much horror, his empathetic nature wasn't able to process all the terrible things. Jonathan didn't want to go back.

One December evening, after a trip with his mom, he came home, gave Daryl a big hug, and, after helping his mom with her luggage, he went outside to the front yard. There, he took his own life with a self-inflicted gunshot wound to the head.

"When I saw Jonathan lying on the ground, I immediately switched into work mode. The police were surprised to find out I was his father; they thought I was too calm. There was no saving him, but I was trying to do everything I could, just as I did on the battlefield.

"Afterward, my wife and I took turns holding each other up. Each of us fell apart at different times, thank God," he said. Daryl tried to consciously process his grief in healthy ways. He never took to the bottle or pills. Instead, he turned to his faith, his family, and to friends. He talked to Jonathan daily.

Yet, he still had nightmares, he still had issues with sleep. He was in physical pain daily due to war injuries, and the face of the man he'd killed would not leave him. So much pain, so much hurt, yet his will to live and to get well was unmatched in anyone I'd worked with so far.

I said, "You need to get these supplements, you are completely depleted."

"Check." He wrote down the names of the supplements.

"You should try mediation and these stress management tools."

Without hesitation, he again agreed, "Check."

"Have you read this? Explored this?"

"Check, check."

But more than coming to us for the answers, he sought them out for himself and brought them back to us. He's the one who said to me, "Have you heard about the term Occupational Stress Injury? It's as a new way of coining PTSD, so we don't feel bad about claiming it."

No, I hadn't, but Canada now uses this term for military and others who have on the job trauma, rather than post-traumatic stress disorder.

"Have you heard of the app Calm, or this program, or this book?"

I was the one taking notes now.

"I tried exposure therapy; it was awful for a few days, but I'm feeling better. It worked for me."

Daryl owned his story; he owned his experiences. He didn't make excuses or apologize or back away from the hard details. He got to work. Very importantly, he involved his wife in every step as his battle buddy, and he kept notes on his progress. He *worked* to get better, showing up for himself and his family at every turn.

I tease Daryl that he is our gold star All Secure student of healing.

Women have become more and more involved in direct combat. From the time I started training with the military in 2013, to meeting the first woman to pass Green Beret selection in 2019, there have been massive strides in allowing females into combat roles. But, to be clear, women have been attached to Special Operations units in various roles for decades. I've met these women and, believe me, I wouldn't fuck with a single one of them.

Kris served in a combat role, intimate with the horrors of war. She was an integral part of her team. Hard as nails, highly motivated, and extremely intelligent, she made for an ideal soldier.

She served with pride and, after a few decades of service, she retired. During a doctor visit on post, she shared the things she was dealing with, the same symptoms the men she served alongside with suffered from, yet the Army doctor told her something that I literally couldn't believe a professional would say: "You can't have combat-related PTSD; you're a woman, and women don't fight in combat, so you can't have PTSD."

This, despite knowing she literally had been in combat. Kris left frustrated, angered, confused, and in tears. It is obvious to anyone with a brain, or a goddamn heart, our women warriors are in need of help and care just as much as the men. Luckily, she was taking steps to help herself by reaching out to us.

For some of our female soldiers, PTSD is brought on by an attack from someone who is supposed to be their brother in arms. Rape and sexual assault are nothing new in the military—one in four women who serve are victims of sexual assault. I met a woman who served in a combat role overseas attached to the Rangers and suffered from war trauma, having witnessed her best friend dying on the battlefield, but also sexual trauma, having been raped by another American soldier. She was nineteen. Leadership swept it under the rug.

Her PTSD was eating away at her insides. When I met her, she was so thin and frail, she looked nothing like the picture of her younger self, fully kitted up, her friend still by her side. Her anger and rage were the biggest things about her, always at a boiling point, oftentimes uncontrollable. The PTSD symptoms she described were exactly those of her male counterparts, yet she wasn't given the same help or respect.

She and her husband, a Special Operations sniper, attended the first All Secure Foundation Special Operations Couples Retreat Workshop. After the final session, she told us how powerful the weekend was for her, to be heard, to learn, to reconnect with her husband. Her face was bright and she was smiling, her physical appearance having changed in just those few days. That's how important it is to know you belong. That's how powerful collective storytelling is. That's how important communication and tools and being part of a tribe are.

She said she hadn't been optimistic about this retreat, believing she'd be on the outside as usual. She thought the other women would bring judgment about her time in service and maybe even the rape, or that she wouldn't have anything in common with them, and that the men wouldn't value her stories because they weren't the same as theirs and that they too would judge her experience of sexual assault. Thankfully, that wasn't the case. As she sat around the fire on the first night, we went around the circle and shared stories. She saw that hers was just as valid as anyone else's.

She left me with something I still hold in my heart—that belonging is powerful and it aided in her healing. She had taken the hard step of reaching out again and asking for help. It had paid off.

We all need a tribe. We all need belonging. And we need to share our stories, to release our pain and emotion, but also to acknowledge the universality of our experiences.

Greg served in Special Operations, a linguist who spoke half a dozen languages, some ancient. He retired after having served around the world, getting to know the people in the places that I had only dreamed about going (especially Egypt, which has been a bucket-list trip for me since I was twelve). He had his fair share of war trauma and complex PTSD.

He called to talk about nutrition, and so we started there, like we do with so many as they first reach out for help. He changed his diet, removing inflammatory foods and fueling his body with badly needed vitamins and minerals. His brain fog lifted, his energy increased, as well as his motivation; his sleep improved, and then his mood lifted.

He was willing to do the work on himself, and it paid off. I can't emphasize enough the critical importance of appropriate sleep, a fundamental component of health and wellness. As he started feeling better and thinking and sleeping better, he could then attack the other issues he was facing. He underwent TMS after seeing Tom share his story on social media about his therapy sessions. He took measurable steps toward healing. When he had a setback, he started to understand that most people often do, and he'd get back to work. In healing complex PTSD, it's often several steps forward and a few back, just as in life.

I am well aware of how easy it would be to breeze through these stories and say to yourself, "So what? I'm not like these people." Maybe you think your story is not as bad, or it's worse. Maybe you think you don't have the strength to mount drastic change in your behavior or choices. Maybe you don't think there's anyone out there willing to help you stay the course.

I'm here to tell you, if you can just get yourself started, take it one small step at a time, you'll see it's doable. You're reading this! You're already doing something for yourself. Keep going.

TWO

Like a Moth to Flame: Depression and Self-Medicating

HE'S DEPRESSED. I MEAN, LIKE A DEEP, BLACK DEPRESSION. If he's not sleeping, he's self-medicating, coming home drunk and passing out on the back porch, finding no place in this "real" world for the warrior he's become.

Who he is now? Not the young person who joined up, all bright-eyed and eager to take on the world, able to sit with his back to a door or not reach for his right hip when a car backfires. He's dark, moody, and lost—though he knows the way to the local drug dealer's house, that's for sure. What a living nightmare.

According to the Department of Veterans Affairs, twenty-two soldiers kill themselves every day. *Twenty-two.* This number includes the veterans, active duty, and reserve. You likely know at least one person who falls into this category. For most, that number is hard to understand. Often, I put it this way: it's more service men and women deaths in a single year than all of the American casualties of the Iraq and Afghanistan war combined.

Can you imagine how we'd respond if over eight thousand kindergarten teachers killed themselves every year? Would we look the other way, like we do with our soldiers?

These are warriors. They are taught to assess problems and remove them. When they feel that they are the problem, they remove the problem. This is the ultimate stressor for every military family—that their soldier will give in and commit suicide.

Add in the large numbers of our populations traumatized by COVID-19, veteran and civilian, and we are looking at an unbelievable spike in PTSD-induced suicides in America.

We have to help them fight to overcome the perception that they can't change, that all is hopeless. It's not.

The first thing you and your PTSD family member need to do? Absorb the biggest message from chapter one: PTSD is a biological condition. Because of this, no matter how tough you are, no matter what kind of battle-seasoned warrior you are, willpower alone will not solve the problem. Yet, it is the perceived lack of willpower that sends the soldier into that dark, sustained depression. They desperately want to stop their bad behavior and terrifying responses to everyday life situations, but they just can't seem to control themselves. They have the fortitude and strength—the willpower—to run into houses filled with bad guys, but back at home, they are horrified to find that they can't stop themselves from hurting those they love. They see themselves as the bad guys now. They are weak and worthless.

But that is so far from the truth. Willpower is bullshit.

Willpower, the Great Mirage

Willpower is a false concept, one that makes us feel like shit for not being able to conquer a challenge or achieve a goal. We've adopted this collective idea that we can just will our way out of something or will our way toward something, even if it means magically fixing a physical problem. Our brain composition and processes are far too complex for that to be the case. Just like you can't heal a torn Achilles with the power of positive thinking, the same is true for damage to the brain.

Don't get me wrong, willpower and positive thinking definitely come in to play when it is time to focus on how to heal, but only in the sense that it can get you through the hard work and long months you will have to put in before you get to a place of health.

For example, I've battled with the same fifteen pounds my whole life: gain, lose, gain, lose. I've always beaten myself up for my lack of strength, or willpower, when it comes to just giving in and eating a couple of cookies and a half bag of chips while vegging out, or not having the willpower to eat sensibly at a restaurant or dinner party. Then the shame cycle will begin in the morning. *Ugh, why the freaking hell did I eat all of that last night?* I judge myself, brushing the crumbs out of my pajamas. Then the shame, oh the shame, for not having the willpower to stop.

Because, again, willpower is bullshit.

Our brains will constantly seek pleasure, comfort, and safety. Have you ever gotten home from work and thought, *Should I go for a run or should I watch reruns of* Sex and the City *while I munch on last night's pizza with a glass of red?* For most of us, our brain will self-sabotage and immediately pick the easy road. You'll find yourself sitting on the couch with Sarah Jessica Parker, cold pizza, a second glass of wine, and a promise to yourself, *I'll run tomorrow.*

Mel Robbins broke this down for us in *The 5 Second Rule.* She understood that the brain will self-sabotage and move toward comfort within five seconds of thinking, *Should I do this or should I do that?* If you don't take action toward the new behavior, like going for a run, your brain within five seconds will talk you into '90s gal-pal TV and a pint of ice cream.

The exact same thing is at play here with PTSD. There is no willpower necessary to change the behavior—you have to have a system and plan in place and then act on that plan. Can change happen overnight? No. It takes time to reach a goal or change a habit, and that time is different for every person.

You can't ignore PTSD and hope it will go away. In fact, research shows PTSD gets worse with time when left untreated, not better.

You can't just stop a behavior because you or your spouse wish it would go away. I hear this on nearly every call from a combat warrior, "Why can't I just stop being angry all the time? Why do I overreact to stupid shit? What's wrong with me? I try to stop, and then it just keeps happening, almost like I'm watching myself do it and I can't control it."

They are angry and deeply depressed. Embarrassed. Ashamed.

Most every call from a spouse, I hear, "Why can't he just stop this behavior? He knows it's wrong, why can't he just stop? He must want to be this way, because no matter how many times I've told him to not be so angry, he just keeps *choosing* to be angry."

If it was that easy, if willpower actually worked to instantly stop aggressive behavior or anger issues, if we could just think something and then flawlessly do that thing every time, the multi-billion-dollar weight loss industry would be bust. We would just will away the weight and make good choices every time.

This is where the biological response comes into play with PTSD.

In your temporal lobe is an almond-shaped mass called the amygdala. This is basically a command center, and one of its operations is a survival mechanism, to make sure you physically respond when a threat is perceived. In stressful situations, the heart pounds, breathing quickens, and spurts of adrenaline wake up the brain and muscles. The fight-or-flight response is activated.

Imagine going through one of those three-story haunted houses with people around every corner to freak you out. Your body jumps and twitches and sweats, ready to run at every noise, punch anything that touches you. Your amygdala has initiated the fight-or-flight response, putting the systems in your body on high alert. Luckily, when you burst out the doors on the other side, still alive and no longer in danger, your heart will return to normal and your brain will slow back down. You'll be exhausted but fine. That kind of tired is called an adrenaline dump—even my husband has nearly passed out asleep after a firefight because of the adrenaline dumping out of his system so quickly.

A soldier has to go through different houses of horror every day for months on end, year after year. The amygdala has been trained to keep the fight-or-flight switch flipped on all the time. The stress response is never allowed to shut down. The soldier does not have any conscious control over shutting down the amygdala, not when he or she is in danger.

Putting you back in that haunted house, think about how you couldn't will yourself to not jump when someone leaped out at you. You might have told yourself, *This time I won't scream*, but if a spiderweb brushed across the back of your neck, you probably shrieked like you were getting macheted. You were jumpy because your brain was constantly looking for threats and reacting. Trying to protect you. Imagine if that threat was *real* and making a mistake could get you or your brothers or sisters in arms killed. A combat brain, unconsciously, is constantly looking for the threat and reacting within a heartbeat of assumed danger. This biological response is why the human race has survived, but it is also responsible for a lot of unnecessary pain and anguish, and eventually depression.

Every story has a beginning, a middle, and an end. Trauma has an end as well, if you can help the brain get there.

One time, I was stopped at a traffic light when another car ran the red, hit me while going over sixty miles an hour, pushing me into the middle of the intersection, where two other cars narrowly missed me. I very nearly died. While awful, the threat was over almost before I knew what was happening.

However, the brain does not perceive that as an ending. Instead, the amygdala has learned that spontaneous threats are around every corner, just like in combat, and will continuously look for that threat to happen again. I couldn't sit at that stop light for months without getting nervous, without grabbing the wheel tightly when cars would come up too fast on me. My amygdala would whisper, *It's unsafe here, get ready for it.* One time a few weeks after the accident, I gripped the steering wheel so tight that Tom asked from the passenger seat, "Why are your knuckles white? Let go!"

Did I consciously respond this way? No. My brain was searching for the end to the story but, with trauma, the brain was stuck in danger-seeking mode. I started to understand why Tom would unconsciously switch lanes under overpasses to avoid snipers or move away from roadkill because one too many times the terrorists had used roadkill to hide bombs. He didn't think, he reacted.

Can you imagine how difficult this can be for someone who has been through multiple combat deployments? Coming home becomes strange and combat zones more comfortable because the brain is familiar now in steps one and two. When the kids freak out over who gets the TV remote, the brain says, *Okay, there's chaos here, I know steps one and two are happening, must protect myself, assess, and shut down the threat. The kids are the threat.* Does that make sense? Not to most of us, but most also aren't living in life-or-death scenarios that require quick, automated decisions.

Anger, violence of action, aggression, hypervigilance, doing tasks exactly as you're trained to do, perfection, regaining control over chaos…these are the tools of combat. These tools become muscle memory. They are used over and over and over again until it becomes the new norm. When the kids are fighting over the remotes, crying and yelling, the dogs are barking, and the mom is getting involved, the brain assesses in seconds that the chaos needs to be controlled, and the muscle memory uses the tools used most often, the same tools used with success overseas.

Anger, violence, perfection-driven aggression. This is training, this is biology, this is not a matter of willing yourself to change.

If we don't start with understanding this, that those suffering from PTSD are not simply weak-willed, then the clinical depression and suicide rate will only continue to rise.

Getting the Warrior to Acknowledge the Depression

Alright, you get it now, willpower alone is not the problem. But what will change the behavior and hopefully end the depression before it goes too dark?

Patience, diligence, willingness to change, and most of all, awareness and planning steps to take when the brain says *threat, react.*

To start, if you can help your person suffering from PTSD to acknowledge the signs of depression in themselves, then maybe they can see the depression as an enemy that needs to be overcome before it gets too strong. The mission is to strike each characteristic of the depression, blast away at the root of it. Focusing on every issue brought on by PTSD at one time is too big. Even focusing on the depression is too big to start with. But if the warrior can make a list of the signs of depression that are being exhibited, then he or she can start developing strategies to combat each one. I think this is a great exercise to do together, but the warrior may not be ready for that just yet. If they are struggling, a therapist can help with creating this list, especially when it comes to helping develop positive strategies. Or just start with baby steps and go to the helpful websites, like the Mayo Clinic's pages on depression.

You know your person best, so you already know some behavior they exhibit that makes you think they are depressed. But let me offer some basic language, maybe put into words stuff you both already know but haven't been able to verbalize. One or all of these can be signs of depression:

- Loss of appetite or eating too much
- Drinking too much, avoiding sobriety/reality
- Taking pills or other drugs to avoid feeling
- Unhealthy weight loss or weight gain
- Overwhelming anxiety over everyday concerns
- Anger or lashing out in response to minor disturbances, or over nothing at all
- Refusing to get exercise or go outside, isolating
- Unable to keep a job
- Unable to finish a project
- Withdrawn, inability to communicate with family or friends
- Fascination with inflicting pain on self
- Reckless behavior
- Suicidal thoughts or statements

This is not a comprehensive list. It can't be; every person is different. But if they could pick just one thing to start working on, what would it be? Again, everyone is different. For Tom, it was his anger.

Sweeping Out the Cobwebs

"Okay," your soldier says, "I'm aware I'm angry. I know I over-react. I hate yelling at my wife, my kids, the dog. I don't want to want to kill the rude guy at the grocery store or the woman driving too fucking slow in the right lane."

Start paying close attention to those triggers. What sets your warrior off? How do they react when they get set off?

Have them picture the kids fighting over the remote, the dogs are barking, the wife starts yelling...they need to picture their response in action: **Stop right there, Soldier. Take a breath. Do not** react. **Remove** yourself from the situation.

They have to have a plan laid out *before* the fit of rage starts, responses that are visualized and then practiced. You have to work together as a couple to decide what you will do when the behavior or triggers happen.

For Tom and me, it was distance. I would walk away, or run, when he would start getting very angry. That only made him angrier and more depressed. We would fight about the fight just as much as what he was mad about in the first place.

Our therapist helped us understand each other and what was happening when he was triggered, and likewise when I was triggered, how to have compassion for each other, and to move away from the situation. We decided when he started to get angry that he would take a break. Our language was, "I'm feeling x, I need to go y." That could be, *I'm feeling angry, or pissed, or hurt, or confused, or whatever, and I need to go for a walk, a drive, to the basement to punch a bag, or in the backyard to catch my breath.* I never pursued him, and he wasn't to pursue me if I asked for the same.

Time allowed for the adrenaline to quiet down and settle. Within ten minutes he was calm, I was calm, and we could then come back together and either speak rationally or ask for more time.

We also have tools for talking to each other. For instance, we promised to never accuse. We will say, "The story I'm telling myself is…," instead of "You did this," or "You did that."

The brain needs to be retrained. Just as you were trained for combat, you have to train for a new life. It takes time, it takes patience, and it is completely doable.

In the meantime, I know it is hard. Very hard. So, let's talk about *your* depression. When your partner, the soldier, returns home as Mr. Hyde, the ugly monster, instead of your sweet and funny Dr. Jekyll, how do you deal with it?

Depression in the Caregiver

It's natural to be frustrated, infuriated, depressed.

I can't begin to put into words the depression and the frustration, the level of hopelessness that comes with loving someone swinging wildly between extreme personalities, who has trauma so deep it seeps into everything. One minute, he's that stable Dr. Jekyll guy, maybe even sweet, thoughtful, loving, funny, charming, and even nurturing but, within a flash, without warning, he's twisted into a rampaging creature.

For Tom, like many combat veterans, he slips into a state like this because he's trying to reclaim order. This is a relentless

Tom, driven to stabilize the world around him. But to me, when I'm just trying to talk to him about a doctor appointment that's been cancelled or that the hardware store didn't have the right size nails, it looks like insanity. If you're "lucky," it's just asshole behavior, like mean-spirited verbal jabs that are completely out of line.

There's little compromising or negotiating with him when he's in this state of mind. He pushes and pushes to the point that I just want to retreat. Retreat into myself. Retreat into my room. Surrender, just to make the chatter stop. But you can't, it's like a dam breaking and there's no way to hold the water back once he gets going. You don't feel safe or secure, there's no rescue in sight, and you know damn well it can get worse. Way worse. There are no time outs. At least, in the beginning for us there weren't. Once he started on something, he would finish it. No matter who he would have to take down in the process, including himself.

What spouse wouldn't be depressed, knowing every morning when you wake up, you're going to have at least three arguments, and likely one that was really going to go south?

The thing is, my warrior always came out the other side of these episodes ashamed. The anger, the rage, the overreaction, the insults—he could hear them coming out of his mouth, but he couldn't stop it. "Sorry," he would say afterward, eyes downcast. But "sorry" lost its meaning years ago. He knew it, and he knew it was his fault. This would put him in a shame cycle that would spiral down into a depression so dark, he might as well have been in Dante's ninth layer of hell. His actions and reactions hurt him as much as me, sometimes more.

People don't realize that or see that, but, as I said before, nothing is more true: hurt people hurt people. *He is hurting, he lashes out. I am hurting now, so he is ashamed. He's embarrassed.* The cycle repeats yet again and feels like defeat. He doesn't like feeling defeated, I don't like to see him defeated. This cycle is continuous and there's little break from it. It's so goddamn heavy, it's so goddamn depressing. When you're in it, you hate it. I even thought I hated him sometimes. I didn't, not really, but the anger in me made me resentful, and it sure felt like hate. Above all else, I just wanted to get back to happy. Always looking for the yellow brick road. *Take us to Oz.* The good witch can wave a wand and make it okay. I tried to be like Dorothy, hoping the ability to change my fate was in a few clicks of my heels and that I could announce to the universe, "There's no place like home." But then home was no longer a sanctuary and, no matter how fabulous those red heels were, they wouldn't get me to where I needed to go. There was no wizard, no magic. This realization made my depression deepen right along with his. *Exactly how long will I be trapped in this tornado?*

Still, I prayed for relief. I begged the universe for answers. *Why me? Why him? Why us? Won't you give his mind, his body, his soul a break? Let the trauma go on a long vacation; in fact, just let it go and never come back.*

I can only get depressed for so long, though. There's no time for it. Anxiety, too. The part of the brain that manages depression also manages anxiety. It is actually quite common for combat spouses to sink into this anxiety-depression cycle. Biology takes over. Like I've said, it's not a matter of willpower.

So, do you have to "fix" your soldier first, before you get to be happy?

No. As a matter fact, stop, take a breath. You need to put on *your* oxygen mask first. The cliché is extremely apt in this instance. You need to get yourself into a healthy enough space that you have the energy and fortitude to save your loved ones and continue to be there for them. The goal is obviously to get them to fight their own depression, but it is easier to help, and to stay safe, if you are able to take deep, nurturing breaths in the process. Here are some things you can do to get the ball rolling in yourself.

Putting Your Oxygen Mask on First

There are many ways to address secondary PTSD and depression in you, the caregiver, from therapy to journaling, but the important thing is to start doing something for yourself. Just jump into it. Baby steps are still steps.

For me, it began with reading constantly. My shelf at home looks like the self-help section of Barnes & Noble. I was arming myself with information and actions to help grow and heal. From Brené Brown to Gabrielle Bernstein, Gary Zukav, Oprah's *Super Soul Sunday* episodes and podcasts, Tony Robbins courses...I was open to anything on how I could grow emotionally and spiritually and better manage my energy and personal health, which was depleted and weakened. Find some books that interest you, step out of your comfort zone—at the end of this book there is an appendix with titles I've found helpful.

Find a friend you can trust, someone with whom you can air out the dirty laundry. I know you love your family and they can be great, but it's also very hard to tell your mama about what your husband did and then go over for Sunday dinner and have everyone sit around the table as if nothing happened. Find someone who won't judge your situation or your partner or steer you to a place you're uncomfortable. It makes all the difference to have a sounding board. I wouldn't have survived without my soul sisters. But just the same, not everything in your home is meant for someone else's ears. Be wise about what you share and with whom. Emotional moments that are between you should stay sacred and private, as long as no one is getting hurt.

See a therapist. Emotionally focused therapy (EFT) and cognitive behavioral therapy (CBT) are both excellent forms of therapy for trauma. Tom and I went through two therapists before we found the right fit. Once we did, I would see her by myself to unload and to deal with my own trauma, along with the weekly couple's sessions. It was a lot of therapy for a year, but it worked and, in part, it saved our marriage.

Journaling is a tried-and-true method for working through issues. There is something about putting pen to paper that helps you see patterns more clearly, helps you see what's working in your life and what's not, where you want to improve and where you're also succeeding. People who journal are more successful with their recovery and tend to be happier. So, write it down.

Take time to do something fun and relaxing just for you. You heard me right, just for *you*. I can hear a collective sigh and an overwhelming feeling that y'all are eye rolling me. *Yes, Jen, great idea, I'll take up a hobby along with managing the house, the kids, my husband, and my job.* But I can promise you this, if you take fifteen minutes a day to do something just for you, you will notice the difference. It could be making sure to get a nice walk in before the kids get up or grabbing a coffee and sitting with a book for twenty minutes a day, joining a yoga class with a friend—just do something that feels good for you. Fill your cup back up. Put that oxygen mask back on.

If you are seriously depressed or suicidal, please, for the love of God, tell someone. Do not wait, get the help you need. Your life is precious, you are loved and needed. Don't wait, seek medical attention immediately.

How to Combat Developing Addictions

Most of us deal with a sliding scale of addictions in our daily lives. We fight with ourselves about eating a third cupcake or opening that second bottle of wine. Addictions are serious, sometimes interfering with an individual's health and sometimes the family around that individual.

Those of us trying to fill dark holes in our psyche are most apt to fall into addictive behavior. Those with PTSD…well, that hole is bottomless. They need someone to throw them a ladder.

But if you're the partner, sitting at home while your spouse is passed out on the pool table at the local watering hole again or you've found your bank account drained from the casino ATM, your desire to help can only last so long. You can throw down that ladder over and over, but you can't make him climb out. The effort to get him to do so is so goddamn tedious and soul-sucking.

It's hard. I get it. But maybe it will help both of you if I can offer some concrete, painless steps to get the process of cleaning up started. And then we can talk about building up the strength to say no to bad habits (drugs, alcohol, adultery) even when times get dark.

I am not an addiction specialist. When I am working with clients, I often refer to the Addiction Center and their website for information and resources. While not a replacement for getting professional help or seeking a doctor's advice on change in diet or behavior, they cover many of the basics I find helpful to share with someone suffering from addiction.

In one of their articles, "4 Steps to Breaking a Bad Habit and Forming a New One" by Jasmine Bittar, updated June 2020, the need to create new habit patterns is highlighted. Bittar discusses various ways in which to make that happen, such as starting with small steps (one beer versus a case) instead of quitting an addiction cold turkey; replacing your old habits with new, healthier ones; and, whenever possible, carefully removing yourself from temptation or friends who may undermine your decision to get clean.

While all of these suggestions seem to be common sense, it's good to hear them, to remind yourself and your loved one that once you make the determination that it's time for a change, it's not rocket science when it comes to finding a pathway to being clean. Yes, it will be hard, but your life and the lives of those you love are worth the hard work.

According to Bittar, who works for Recovery Worldwide, "Fighting the need to use or give in to your habits can be very exhausting [...]. Love yourself enough to stop doing damage to your present and future."

Though it will be difficult for some to hear, you or your loved one will also most likely need help moving away from those self-defeating habits. Addiction dependency must be battled on a biological level as much as a mental and emotional level, which is why so many addicts are only able to kick their habits after intervention and rehab, and then maintain sobriety with continued support from professionals or the community. Luckily, there is a lot of addiction help out there. I highly recommend starting with a visit to a physician, who can assess how much damage has been done by drugs, alcohol, or unprotected sex. I know those are not easy conversations, finally admitting to your doctor, "Yeah, when I said two drinks a day last time, I really meant one to two bottles." No matter how embarrassed you feel, you can deal with the momentary shame. Information is imperative when it comes to creating a full-fleshed action plan.

Remind the addict: You can do it. You have been in control of your body and mind before, you can do it again.

THREE

#Nofilter: Anger, Aggression, and Violence

IT SEEMS OBVIOUS WHY ANGER, AGGRESSION, AND VIOLENCE come into play with complex PTSD, especially regarding people who have combat trauma.

When Tom entered the army, he left the bubble that most of us live in, where we stroll around our neighborhoods or bike blithely down main street, waving at neighbors and watching out for cars—but it doesn't cross our mind to be on the lookout for a kid strapped into a suicide-bomb vest. In order to prepare for the "real" world of war, Tom was trained to save others and survive. Trained to be physically, mentally, and emotionally aggressive. He was trained to be angry, he was trained to be violent. You don't go to war and hug a terrorist; you go to war and you kill a terrorist. You don't go to war and have a tea party with someone who's trying to bomb a subway station in London; you put a hot frying pan to his head until he talks. You sacrifice your sense of morality in order to save people.

Every bit of that ugliness comes back home with that soldier.

Tom, like all the men and women in the armed forces who've served overseas, has lived outside the bubble, and there's no getting back in. When he came home, he understood something he hadn't before: our safety is a construct.

We aren't safe, not even here—something terrible can happen at any second. There are bad people among us who don't play fair or nice. They kill children. They use their wives to walk into a crowded market with an unpinned grenade. When a twelve-year-old approaches with an AK, Tom knows that the kid's bullets are just as deadly as an adult's, and he has to decide if he saves the life of the child or his troops.

For most of us at home, drinking coffee with our feet up, righteously monologuing about how we would never kill someone, especially a child…we do not have the faintest idea about the truth of the world. Do you think our soldiers, our young men and women who have gone to war for us, who are doing what we asked of them, do you think they joined up so they could face down a child?

You know who wants peace more than you? A soldier.

Instead, after realizing how horrific it can be outside the bubble, they come home hoping to regain that sense of peace and safety, only to find that their brain just won't "forget" what happened. What they did. What they had to do, for us, to keep our bubbles whole.

So many reasons for them to be angry, both emotionally and biologically. Sadly, only a very few have the tools to dismantle their rage on their own. That's where we step in. Let's give them the tools and help them learn how to save themselves.

I know, I know, it's easy to say—but I do know what I'm talking about. I've seen the strongest men and women toil and crack under the burden. I've lived with the shitshow that is PTSD. I still have days, even with Tom as aware and careful as a loving, strong man can be, when I think: *Will this ever end? When can I have my husband back? Not even like he was before he went into the service, that ain't gonna happen, not ever, but at least a little of him.*

I know that Tom is changed, and we have this Tom now to love and to help heal. I get that, but sometimes I just want the Tom back from fifteen minutes ago, prior to the laundry "not being done right" and him taking a swing at the wall. The one who was dancing with me in the kitchen, laughing and poking fun. Making me feel light and loved. There was a kiss and a hug, a long one. The kind that made me sink right into his skin. The kind that I didn't want to break from. Ever.

I want that back. For fuck's sake, it was fifteen minutes ago. But now I am hurt, he's ashamed. Here we are again. His perfection-driven aggression is the hardest of all the symptoms for me. It causes self-doubt, makes me think maybe I'm the one in the wrong. It breaks apart my self-love. It tears at my self-confidence.

Relentless, compulsive, nonstop picking at me. His brain has been rewritten to see all things as a threat, and chaos means he needs to get control or die. That same boots-on-the-ground mindset is applied to unfinished household chores or yard work or anything that seems not in line.

"Get in line, soldier." That's how he responds to me now.

"I am *not* your *soldier!*" The countless times I've told him that. "Stop barking at me! I don't take orders from you. You're talking to me like a private. I am not one of your brothers. I am not one of your subordinates. I am not a terrorist. I am not a threat."

I am not your soldier.

I am the protector of your heart. I am the guardian of your spirit. I am the healer. The helper. The lover. The soulmate. The best friend. The comic relief and the strong shoulder to bear the weight with you.

I am not your soldier.

Don't treat me this way. Why can't you see who I am? Why don't you know this by now?

Why am I still here...?

How could I leave?

He is my heart. My lover. My best friend. My soulmate. My sanity-check. My comic relief. My pillar of strength. My teacher. My everything.

When Anger Rules the Roost

Sometimes I wish I could put a filter on his mouth. But when anger shows its ugly head, all bets are off, there's no filter for what he's putting down.

The anger or aggressive behavior that shows up unannounced and at the most inconvenient times not only causes him to spiral, but I can spiral out right along with him if I'm not careful. As I've said, I'm a laid-back kinda girl at heart, and it takes an awful lot to get me spun up...but when combating anger and aggression daily, it wears on you, it gets to you, it...well, it makes you angry. There have been times when I can see the buildup happen within Tom, the physical and emotional charges being set off, and I know what's coming. Perhaps it's the knowing that's so unnerving. Like, if I'm enduring another lecture on how to properly load the dishwasher, I know it will inevitably lead to a full-out raging battle, whether or not I'm participating. He can launch into a fit of anger even if unprovoked or over seemingly very insignificant things, and my reaction doesn't seem to matter. I've tried them all, to remain quiet and small, or go big and angry, anything so he will shut up and the battle will be over. Not won, just over.

He's shifted into the warrior mindset (the same mindset that is an asset in combat), that they must win at all costs because losing a battle means death. Winning, overcoming, pushing past comfortable, doing unimaginable shit to deal with the situation at hand. Fight. No freeze, no flight. Just fight until it's over. Fight until it's won.

This response to danger is necessary. This response to mundane, everyday issues is toxic. It is dangerous. It leads to a lot of WTF moments. Not just in my mind, but in his, as well, when he comes back to himself.

I mentioned earlier that my wedding night was a pivotal moment in our relationship. A make-or-break moment. A WTF, terrifying moment.

Let me start by saying surprises are a huge trigger for Tom, as they are for most people with PTSD. When we found out that the wedding we had been planning for the following year had to happen in eight days, because we were trying to buy a house together and the VA required us to be married to get the home loan, Tom struggled to roll with the changes. I didn't realize it at the time, but for him, having to work out moving details, incoming family details, and ceremony details on the fly was too much. To me, he just seemed out of sorts and distant. I thought maybe he was not wanting to marry me. But no. I didn't know it yet, but his warrior-alter-ego Crawler was taking over, to help put order to the chaos in Tom's head.

Our wedding ceremony on Tybee Island consisted of the two of us, a photographer, and an officiant. The rain had cleared the beach, and we had a gorgeous sunset to ourselves. The vows we wrote to each other were heartfelt. I felt like we were the only two people in Savannah. In the world. It was perfect.

After our simple ceremony, we had dinner and then went barhopping with a group of friends. By the second bar, I was asking Tom to slow down. I encouraged his friends to stop ordering drinks. Instead, Tom was getting mad at me, and soon enough, he was ignoring me. At a crowded and popular downtown Savannah rooftop bar, he sat at a table alone with the wife of a friend, a self-proclaimed Barbie. I tried a couple of times to get him to dance, or at least talk to me, but there was no having it. Instead, he was at that table for two hours, in a drunken conversation I was not part of. On our wedding night.

I finally had enough of being ignored and asked him to come back to the hotel with me; it was late, and the bar was closing up. He was blackout drunk, slurring and stumbling as we made our way back. I was hurt beyond belief. I should have known, for my own sake, to wait until he was sober before calling him out. Yet, the tidal wave of disappointment only grew the more I thought about it. I was crushed and pissed off. I'd had a few drinks myself, and so out came the hurt, pouring onto the streets of downtown Savannah.

"Do you realize you didn't even dance with me on our wedding night? Or talk to me, for that matter? Why did you spend the entire night with *her*?"

As we got closer to the hotel, he snapped. For a second, he'd simply been embarrassed, ashamed of himself…but embarrassment was a massive trigger for Tom's anger. His face twisted into a mask of rage, his eyes a solid black. When we walked into our hotel suite, he grabbed my shoulders and then pushed me, hard, so that I fell onto to the tile floor. He was throwing things, screaming that he'd made a mistake, he should have never married me. Crawler had shown up and he was going to take control of the situation, do what it took to win. He shoved me around, screaming in my face. Thank God he didn't punch me. I don't think I'd be here today if he had. His body was trained to respond and kill. That wasn't lost on me then, and it still isn't lost on me. Or him.

I was packed and ready to leave Tom by the time he woke up the next morning. He didn't remember what had happened the night before. He didn't remember the last bar we'd been at, or the walk home, or the fight. He thought we merely got into a little wordplay. You know, exchanged a few hard words.

When I showed him my bruised arms…his face, I'll never forget. Shock, disgust, and embarrassment contorted his features. He jumped out of bed and fell to his knees in front of me. "Please God, please tell me it wasn't me that did that to you!"

I looked at Tom, disturbed that not only could he hurt me like this, but also that he didn't remember.

He knew he'd made a big mistake and deeply regretted it; the despair came off of him in waves. He begged me to forgive him. How could I? He'd stolen so much from me.

He understood. In that moment, he didn't want me to stay, to see him that way. He stumbled to his feet and told me to go, urging me toward the door, overwhelmed with shame and horror.

On our way back to his apartment, Tom asked if we could go back to the site of our vows. I agreed, half-reluctant, half-longing for a do-over. We sat on "our" bench as we called it, a place at the end of the beach that we'd gone many times to watch the sunset. Now, we were once again staring off into the horizon, but it felt as if we were miles apart. He asked if he could hold my hand.

"Not yet."

It was the only thing I said for two hours.

Finally, he asked, "Are you going to leave me? I don't blame you if you want to, if you need to. It might be better if you do, I'm too broken."

Instead, I turned into him, wrapped my arms around him. "I'm not leaving. But I will next time. If it even looks like you're thinking of raising a hand to me, or throwing shit around, I'm out. But that's not what I want." I'd drawn my line in the sand, and he knew it was real.

We didn't talk about it again, not then. It was too big. I was willing to fight out of it. But unless he started showing up, unless he started fighting for us, too, and went to therapy starting Monday morning, I was done.

On Sunday, I had to fly back to St. Louis. I had two friends check on him. I was terrified he was going to kill himself out of shame. They took the alcohol out of his house, took his guns. For a warrior, that's not an easy thing, letting someone take your guns. It is absolutely critical, however. If someone is at risk of suicide, you remove the weapons.

I ask spouses all the time: Is he willing to get the help he needs? Is he willing to put down the bottle? Is he willing to go to therapy and try healing modalities? No? Well, then, what are you going to do? You cannot make someone want to get better, they have to want it for themselves.

That Monday, Tom did start the anger management therapy. It was his decision, but we both thought that's what this was. Anger issues. Unfortunately, this is how PTSD is usually uncovered—when someone's anger spins out of control. At least he was finally on the path to discovering he had PTSD.

Tom wanted to save us. He got to work on himself. But it wasn't as if the night after our wedding Tom decided he wasn't going to have PTSD anymore and so, snap, all of a sudden, he was normal again. No, he had twenty-five years of death and loss and destruction and ugliness woven into his psyche; it was going to take a lot of time to unravel what had been so tightly sewn.

Once he understood what was happening, though, that he suffered from severe complex PTSD, he worked even harder. He never made an excuse, or if he did, he corrected himself. He never missed an appointment. He never said, *I don't want to try,* or *I don't want to go.* He fought for us just as much as he fought for himself.

It was a solid year of help before the real Tom emerged. The alcohol abuse stopped and the threats of physical violence stopped.

He worked on himself 24/7. When he understood how it was Crawler, not Tom, who had shown up on our wedding night, it made it easier for him to forgive himself, and for me to forgive him. It hadn't been Tom that night. Because of his work and determination, I know Crawler won't show up in that way again.

We Are Not Alone

It's not just a handful of people dealing with being scared in their own home, knowing their loved one needs help before he or she hurts someone. I think you know you're not alone, yet I also know how big it feels, to have to stand up to an aggressor who you happen to love and don't want to see in jail.

It's true, everyone's story is different, but let me offer a few more examples of homes under duress, so you can see the universality and the hope.

I recently had a call with a Ranger named Jim, thirty-two years old, home from his fourth deployment and countless training exercises, schools, and combat. His last rotation was a bitch. He came home to a wife and three kids, all of whom had noticed a shift in his behavior after his second deployment, when he lost two of his men. This time, they were met with a man who they barely recognized. There were now no light moments when he was around. No loving moments.

"Sometimes I just get so angry," said Jim, "like raging angry, and I don't know why. I don't know where it comes from. When I start yelling at my wife or getting short with my kids, I feel like it's an out-of-body experience, like I'm standing there watching me say what I'm saying but it's not coming from me. I can't stop saying awful things, even though all I'm thinking in that moment is *shut the fuck up, just stop.* But I can't. I don't know why, and I don't know what's wrong with me. I am too screwed up now. They would be better off without me."

He didn't mean that he wanted to end his life. What he meant was that the man he trained to be and the man who was required to fight overseas isn't the kind of man that his family should have to live with. He didn't know how to be both, a killer overseas and a cuddler at home.

It doesn't work that way, at least for most. The switch doesn't just flip after a flight home, from battle to bedroom; the brain doesn't function in that manner. All too often, I get calls from warriors on the edge because willpower, which they have in spades when in the field, doesn't work for shit at home. Yet, for some reason, we believe that we can will our bodies and brains to perform the way we want them to, to re-rewire the rewiring without any help.

This type of anger and aggression isn't an issue that will simply go away with time or something to just overpower. If you admit that you're feeling off and not quite right, it does not mean you're weak or you're not able to perform the tasks at hand. That simply isn't true.

I asked my Ranger client, "Would you rather go into battle with someone who is physically fit, who has taken the time to shoot on the range daily so he is an excellent marksman, who has gone through the schools and completed the training, who is getting sleep, and eating right, and is mentally and emotionally strong, *or* would you rather go into battle with someone who is still training, still going through all of the schools, still shooting daily but also drinking himself to sleep, which is only three to four hours of crappy sleep, who is taking uppers and downers, is eating like shit, and hasn't dealt with mental and emotional issues that are likely clouding his thought process, and worst of all, who is on the edge of a complete breakdown?"

Jim picked the first one. They all pick the first one.

Being a warrior means you are physically fit, emotionally fit, mentally fit, and spiritually fit. To be the best at what you do, no matter what, that is what a warrior does, so you have to work on and improve your emotional, mental, and spiritual game when you're faltering. The bottom-line truth is that being a strong warrior means asking for help, no matter what kind of help that is, so that you can do your job to the very best of your ability.

Jim's anger problem is the problem of thousands of warriors, as well as spouses with secondary PTSD, and others combating PTSD. Jim isn't an asshole, he doesn't mean to act the way he acts, and yet he does. This causes a shame-and-guilt response, which for many warriors, leads to drinking or isolation to cope with feeling out of control.

I'm going to talk about isolationism in a later chapter, both for the warrior and for the spouse, but it is important to note that warriors, just as much if not more than civilians with PTSD, do not want their personal stuff out there. Because of this reticence for anyone to see them as less than a competent warrior, they usually ask the spouse to remain quiet. Danger gets hidden behind a veil of secrecy and shame.

If the community looks away from inappropriate behavior, or even encourages destructive behavior, then they are part of the problem. As individuals, we need to step up and intervene if necessary. This includes a brother in arms.

One time when Tom and I were teaching PTSD resiliency at Ft. Bragg to a group of Green Berets, I asked them, "If you're on the battlefield and one of you gets shot, do you do triage and drag him to safety, or do you just let him bleed out and die?"

They stared at me, silently. I said, "Come on, raise your hand if you are on the battlefield and you would do anything to save the person to your left or right?"

Every single hand raised.

"Okay, that was obvious, right?" I paced the room filled with 450 soldiers. "I get it. You don't need to raise your hand for this next one, but I do want you to mentally raise your hand. How many of you have stood by and watched one of your buddies get into a bar fight, or flip out on someone for no reason, or know they are constantly in a state of anger or aggression at home? How many of you watch as a buddy is drinking the bar dry, night after night? How many are watching as pills are popped to get up or to take it down? How many have watched or encouraged your buddy to hook up with a girl even though he's married?"

I looked around the room, letting it sink in.

"If you were raising your hand, then you are allowing your buddy to bleed out on the battlefield. You're not helping him by staying silent—you're loading the gun."

You could hear a pin drop, along with a few heads.

My intention is never to judge or to shame someone, but I feel it is imperative to create awareness, to help open eyes to the problems that plague the community, to the culture that kills. To continue to turn a blind eye to the anger, aggression, and reckless behavior at home is turning away from a situation that can go from bad to worse in a blink of an eye.

Tom has had friends, elite warriors, badasses who were beyond capable in every aspect of their job, come home and really hurt their spouse in a fit of rage or injure their children. A few have killed their wives. Those men are now dead. They almost always committed suicide immediately after the act was done and the rage evaporated.

We know there are as many reasons for suicide as there are people. Veterans and their reasons can vary widely, but, most often, statistical research shows that a high number of suicides do happen after a family argument or disruption. If we can look at how anger and aggression fuel the disruption, and we work on removing anger from the home, then we are also actively working to reduce veteran suicide, while also giving them tools to achieve a better quality of life.

What You Can Do

As you know from Tom's story, there is hope, linked to concrete steps you can take.

I reminded Jim and his wife that PTSD is a biological response, describing the physical and emotional trauma and how that impacts his brain—his thinking, sleeping, interactions—and that what he was going through was a very typical response. Most importantly, with proper healing modalities, he can get to the other side of it. That there was no need to isolate or leave his family.

That they wouldn't be better off without him in their life.

Of course, not everyone is like Tom. PTSD affects each person differently, to varying degrees. A biological need for personal safety always, always has to come first, and any sense of safety insecurity can short-circuit the PTSD trip wire. While my career is focused on helping to save warriors and their relationships, I've also worked with many civilian spouses who were being abused, whose partners were in complete denial and wouldn't get the help they needed and, so, would get physical from time to time, especially when drinking or doing drugs. To every person in this position, military or civilian, I say the same thing: get out and get safe. And when the partner starts getting the help they need, and they start taking the hard steps involved in self-improvement, then you can consider returning. Physical violence is never an acceptable resolution, whether it's a male or female doing the abusing. Get yourself and your kids out of the house and allow for that person to heal in the way that they need, or you need to move on, because all of us deserve safety and a good life, no matter how much we love our warrior.

Besides keeping yourself safe, what else can you do if you're dealing with this in your house?

- Get professional counseling. I can't stress this enough. Most people aren't meant to fight this battle alone, and you shouldn't have to. Tom and I turned our lives and relationship around with the help of a seasoned trauma and marriage therapist, who we saw weekly for over a year and still see monthly. You don't need to wait for things to get so bad that there is no turning back. I'll never forget when my mom, in shock, asked why we were in marriage therapy. I said, "Because I want to stay married." We didn't wait until we were completely broken; we went when the cracks started to appear. Now, we go to check in with our growth.

- Those with PTSD must come up with a plan for how to handle the anger but do so during a period of calm. Fits of rage don't usually go hand-in-hand with logic. Rational solutions and procedures need to be decided on ahead of time. All parties involved should be calm and, together, come up with techniques they can use when the anger does show up. As a matter fact, those techniques should be practiced. Roleplay out an angry scene, you'll see what I mean. If you can visualize the techniques in action, it will be easier to fall back on them in moments of high emotion.

- Get space. Take a break. However, what sounds like a simple technique can become very challenging during an outburst, so you have to commit to taking this type of action when you're not triggered. Train yourself to take a break from the argument and go for a walk, or run or work out, play guitar, write it down, punch a bag… you get the idea. Create space between the two of you. Both must agree to not discuss the topic again until all heads are clear and calm. If that means you need to wait twenty-four hours before bringing it up again, then do that. One caveat: if you can't talk about it calmly, then address it with your therapist first.

- If you have PTSD, you need to identify your triggers and write them down. You should be keeping a journal, which helps tremendously to catch your patterns. When you notice something bothering you, write down what happened in detail—you don't have to write a big essay, bullet points work just as well. When you start to create awareness of what's happening and your reactions, it will be easier to come up with plans on how to avoid those triggers or deal with them in a constructive manner.

- Include your spouse or partner: ask them what triggers they've noticed, and be clear in what you need from them in order for you to avoid them. For example, if you get triggered by an entryway that is always overflowing with backpacks and shoes and coats, that means all it takes to start the process of becoming agitated and angry is for you to walk in the door and see the mess. That is a trigger you need to address. And now that you are conscious of it, you might ask your spouse and kids to help keep that area clean and explain why you need it that way. "Hey, when I come home after a stressful day at work, I walk in the door and see clutter, which sets me off. I can't handle clutter well because of my training and it makes me feel anxious, so if you can each keep this area neat, it really will help my process of adjusting to my environment." Caveat: keep in mind that life sometimes is messy and no one or family is perfect, so it can take a while to find and understand all your triggers.

- You have to be your own advocate. Seek out advice from professionals who work with anger management, even if your first step is to google TED Talks on anger or read books on how to constructively manage outbursts. You have to search and research to find and discover what works for you, for your family, and then you have to do it and you have to do it daily. Otherwise, it's like saying, I'm going to run a marathon. I've never run a day in my life, but you know what? I'm gonna put on my tennis shoes once in a while and see how far I get....Well, you're not going to get far in a marathon, that's for sure, not if you're training haphazardly. If you want to get healthy, you've got to get up every morning and you have to be dedicated to that goal, and your goal should be: I'm gonna live a life that I deserve, which is to be emotionally, mentally, and spiritually okay.

• With anything in life, applying tools takes time. There is no shortcut to getting there. Tom and I didn't get control of anger outbursts on the first or the thirtieth try; it's something we consciously worked on daily for over a year and, from time to time, still need to address. Change your perception about self-awareness, make it a lifetime habit to check in with yourself and make course corrections if necessary.

• This bears repeating: If violence is at play in the relationship, then the first step for the spouse is to find a secure, safe place. If that means calling 911, then you need to do that, for both of your sakes. Too many spouses have been seriously injured or killed in a fit of violence, especially when alcohol is involved. If you do not have anyone to turn to but need a place to go, and you're not willing to call 911, call the local hotlines for guidance or drive directly to a woman's shelter, where they are set up to protect you. Once you and any children are safe, and your immediate needs are covered, you need to quickly seek professional help for you and your loved ones.

Understand Yourself(selves)

I've mentioned Tom's alter ego, Crawler, a few times. Understanding this "different self" offered Tom and I a life rope, and likely had the biggest impact on how we deal with the anger and aggression when it comes up.

It was my therapist who first presented this particular concept of various selves in a way that clicked and connected with me so deeply that I could feel it on a spiritual level. Stacey told me about a therapy practice regarding personalities, which is called Parts of You. There is a lot of research out there on multiple personalities developing in people who need to protect themselves, usually from some very extreme trauma in childhood; now, put that into the context of your own life and think about how your personality changes on a subconscious level when you're around different people or in different situations. I'm not talking about the extremes of what we would refer to as a personality disorder, but we do have different sides of ourselves that we call up to present to the world at any given time. Stacey pointed out that I'm not the same Jen when I'm around my girlfriends on a Friday night versus when I'm at a board meeting (and, boy, ain't that the truth). When I'm working with my kids, doing homework or telling bedtime stories, I'm not the same person as I am when I'm alone with my husband—especially when we are being intimate. Only Tom sees that Jen, but we both like her.

In regards to responding to anger and aggression, when I'm feeling really mousy and small because I'm afraid either physically or emotionally, I understand now that the part of me I call Jenny has come forward. Jenny is me as an eight-year-old girl, a child who'd been bullied mercilessly for years at home and at school and felt unloved, ugly, dumb, insignificant, and desperate for someone to love her while believing she was deeply unworthy.

Jenny shows up in my life when I'm feeling unworthy or unloved, and I now know why sometimes, in those moments, I act out like an eight-year-old, powerless or just plain childish. This is the part of me who shows up when I'm feeling really insecure, maybe fixating on whether or not I'm pretty enough, skinny enough, smart enough. "No, I'm not!" says Jenny from a corner in my mind. "I'm not good enough for Tom, he's going to leave me." So then, I'll start moping over nothing, acting childishly, and being illogical, and Tom will walk in the door. Out of nowhere (as far as he's concerned), I'll say, "Are you interested in someone else?"

However, when I am projecting confidence, a strength that I feel in my bones, and everything's kind of going right and I'm leading the charge, well, that's Jenna. Jenna is my warrior, the part of me who pushes through all the tough shit, who shows up in the hard moments, turning away from fear because she's determined, she's loyal, she's self-sacrificing. When I can tap into that strength, I'm Jenna. But if I'm feeling overwhelmed and scared, my reactions are more that of Jenny.

Day-to-day, though, I'm pretty much just Jen. I'm usually laid-back. I love my family, and other people, and going to new places. I'm creative and adventurous, drama-free. That's Jen.

That's me most of the time. I'm sure there are more parts, but these are the easily identifiable parts of me that either come from past trauma or past strength.

When I talked to Tom about Parts of You, he had the same kind of light-bulb moment.

We dug in and talked about who he was, about the multiple sides of him that came together to create the whole. One of the greatest ah-ha moments came when we identified his anger, his violence, and his rage as his warrior self. That part of him we named Crawler, after his call sign, Nightcrawler.

We were able to identify how, when Tom was in his warrior mindset, it was the Crawler part of him calling the shots, and he was powerful and not easy to shake. He had been developed out of life-and-death necessity. Crawler was not day-to-day Tom; there was an actual physical, emotional, and spiritual shift that occurred in Tom when he was triggered and became Crawler, and it had been happening on a completely subconscious level.

Plain old Tom doesn't like dishes in the sink, but he'd rinse them out, mutter under his breath, put them away, and go on with his day. But if he was triggered, then Crawler showed up, noticed the cups in the sink, and lost his shit. Crawler needed the "chaos" in front of him to be quashed and, so, became belligerent and stern, letting the "troops" know with an angry voice or manner that this would not be tolerated. If I lashed back (because it's damn hard not to) or cowered away, then I wasn't responding like a soldier.

It was never about the dish in the sink. Any perceived disrespect, especially in his world of order and rank, can send Tom packing and Crawler swiftly moving to the forefront of the issue.

Crawler would become aggressive, trying to maintain control of the dishes, and me, slamming things on countertops before raging down the hallway.

Now, armed with the understanding that Crawler was taking over, Tom could often identify what was happening, shake his head, and go, "Yeah, yeah, that's totally what happens when I become Crawler, I lose Tom. I don't react or think or love or behave like Tom. I think and react like a warrior." An epiphany for him came with understanding that *a warrior wasn't needed in that moment.*

I didn't need one of America's most elite soldiers to have a conversation with me about how to do the dishes. I did need Tom there, though, my partner. I needed Tom to help around the house or help with the kids or help with work.

We spent a lot of time talking about Crawler and his place in this world—and how we both are grateful for Crawler and that there are men and women like Crawler who go to battle for us.

While calling attention to these dark parts of ourselves, there was no judgment. We agreed never to use this knowledge disparagingly or to harm or hurt each other. That is *extremely* important. I never say, "Well, fuck you, Crawler." Or "I wish Crawler would die and never come back." Crawler is a part of Tom, just like the impish side of him we call Tommy is a part of Tom, and Tom is the man I love and respect. The whole Tom.

So much of healing with PTSD is creating awareness around the situation and then creating a path to a healing solution. Once again, my Tom dug in and did work on himself, trying to decipher when and why Crawler would appear, and then what to do with him when he did. He didn't scoff or laugh at the concepts or the process, he just went for it.

At one point, in a therapy session, Stacey asked him if he'd be willing to take part in an uncomfortable exercise.

Tom leaned forward with a smirk, alert. "What the fuck, let's do this."

She pointed to an empty chair in the corner of her office. "Can you take Crawler—that anger, that part of you—and remove it from yourself for just a moment and put it in the chair across from you? Can you put Crawler in that chair, away from you, so you have some space from him?"

We got quiet for a minute and Tom really took that Crawler personality and he pulled it out of himself. An imagined Crawler sat across from him—a young, fit, tough-as-balls soldier. I could see from his face, this was real for my husband.

"Who is he, Tom? Who is that sitting across from you? Describe him."

It took Tom a few seconds to answer. "He's an elite warrior. He's highly trained, he's deadly. He's really good at getting information out of the bad guys. Any means necessary. He's a loyal and dedicated soldier. He will do whatever it takes to get the job done." He paused but went on. "He will use whatever measures of violence and aggression that it takes to get the job done. He's dark, like a shadow. But he's me."

"What do you want to say to Crawler?"

Tom broke down. Choking out his words, he looked at Crawler and said, "Thank you. Thank you for keeping me alive."

Then I was sobbing, too, because it was true. Crawler had an immense purpose in this life. He'd kept my Tom alive and saved hundreds, maybe thousands, of innocent lives.

But Crawler's time was over. It was done. Crawler was no longer necessary for survival. Tom was retired now, no longer active overseas. Crawler did not need to show up in our marriage anymore or in Tom's relationships with his child or stepchildren. His part in Tom's life was done.

Tom thanked Crawler again. He thanked him for keeping him alive. And doing what it took to keep others alive. And for doing the things that most humans can't even imagine doing in order to keep our country safe. We both thanked him. We both honored Crawler.

After twenty-five years of training and muscle memory, it's not like Crawler just—poof—disappeared. He shows back up, trying to take control, and he's not polite about it. But at least we can now identify who it is showing up. This knowledge and method of therapy has been one of the single greatest points of healing for Tom, to be able to see Crawler, to thank him, to honor him, to respect him, to not judge the choices that he made, to accept what he did while Crawler, to forgive himself for unthinkable things he's done, and to tell Crawler thank you and it was time for him to retire.

So, what did we do with this information? First of all, we agreed beforehand that my strategy for dealing with Crawler would be for me to say, "Crawler's here," or "I don't need Crawler to complete this task." I am consciously not rude or condescending. I am simply recognizing the part of his personality that shows up and yet isn't necessary to complete the task at hand.

My exceptional husband has also developed the ability to recognize his shift in personality, to acknowledge when Crawler has stepped forward. For the most part, he is able to shut Crawler down and walk away until he is back in control.

This is the single greatest tool that we have come across in managing the anger in our house. Tom began using other modalities, too, and maybe this tactic wouldn't have worked so well if he wasn't taking care of his mental health and his body in other ways. My gut feeling, however, is that this is the big gun in our arsenal.

FOUR

Booze, Women, and Adrenaline: The Reckless Behavior

RECKLESS BEHAVIOR IS BORN AT A SUBCONSCIOUS LEVEL. IN MY early twenties, after the childhood trauma and then the brutal sexual trauma, I never stopped and thought, "Hey, I'm partying, out of control, I'm making bad decisions…I must have PTSD."

I wouldn't have acknowledged I was reckless, much less ever associated with a diagnosis that was hardly mainstream in the '90s. That was also true in the military community. It wasn't like the guys I was working with, whether they were contractors or active duty, were walking around saying, "Oh hey, I have reckless behavior. It must be because of my PTSD, I should do something about that." They'd heard of combat trauma, but no warrior was ever going to admit that maybe he was out racing motorcycles at 150 mph or drinking until blacking out or even playing Russian roulette because the violence and death he'd been part of overseas was messing with his head.

Instead, dangerous behavior has been culturally normalized in the military. No one is questioning recklessness. *Eh, he's just doing what warriors do, they're tough.* He just drank a fifth and then went after a biker dude for standing too close? Why wouldn't he, he's a badass.

PTSD has been stigmatized as a disorder for the weak-minded. Recklessness can't be a symptom of PTSD, the soldiers want to believe, because "No one who is sick has the bravery, the mental fortitude, and the strength that I have. I'm not weak. I don't have combat trauma, I signed up for this. I've volunteered to go back three times. Ten times. And look at me now, I'm brave. I can do anything to anyone. I'm invincible. Though, really, I just don't care if I die."

When I met Tom, he was in the thick of reckless behavior. At that time, I didn't realize he did not care if he lived or died. That is true of many people with complex PTSD. Part of Tom's behavior was really him asking the universe to end it for him so he didn't have to.

ALL of Us Have Choices

As we began to hang out more, my own reckless behavior kicked right back into full swing. We were two trains, going a million miles an hour. A collision was bound to happen, but I was working in a community of train wrecks, it wasn't just us. It was everyone on the training missions, the other contractors, the role-players, and our clients, the Seals or Green Berets or

Rangers. Most everyone was a fucking train wreck and thought living on the edge was expected of them. It was normal to be reckless. It was what we did. For us, that usually looked like just really heavy drinking. There was rarely a night we weren't drinking the bar clean, a behavior I'd stopped indulging in fifteen years ago. I ended up becoming a wreck all over again—though I never did that kind of drinking around my kids. I was living two completely different lives, being one Jen when I was away on military exercises and another Jen when I was home.

I think for our soldiers that's what it's like. I get the attraction of deploying, I get the attraction of training and going on these missions for weeks on end, doing something important, and not having to curb my behavior while I'm doing that important thing. I get why the guys are like, "It's easier for me to be gone." You're not dealing with the house or the kids or the bills or school projects or football games that run at the same time as dance lessons or a nagging mother-in-law or a leaky faucet. When you're deployed, it is required that you focus 100 percent on your duty to country and leave family problems behind. You have a situation where people are working fifteen or sixteen hours a day, four or five days a week, often under stressful work conditions. So, in order to decompress, the tribe goes to the bar, drinking from noon until two in the morning, trying to have fun and forget all the horrible shit. Anything goes. The majority are making bad choices or poor choices, some more than others, some worse than others.

When Tom and I were first together, we'd often go out and party with Teddy, one of Tom's Army buddies. The guy could drink, but he certainly didn't stand out in that regard. He had the biggest heart of anyone I knew and was always entertaining to be around, being silly or pulling crazy stunts. What we didn't know was that he was also addicted to heavy drugs. We had no idea he was using heroin, meth, coke...any drug he could get his hands on, anything to stop from thinking and feeling. One night, he called and confessed to Tom he had been doing everything he could to take himself out without doing the actual act.

He would sit in his garage with a shotgun in his lap every night, getting drunk, getting high, and trying to figure out if he should pull the trigger that night or wait another day—with his two kids and his wife inside. When you have no love for yourself or respect for yourself, you can't have it for others. I cannot say that enough. It wasn't that he was being selfish, it was that he couldn't question what he was doing because he was so buried in trauma that he literally couldn't see anything but black despair surrounding him. He couldn't see that his decisions were affecting others. It's not that he was stupid; on a logical level, he could tell himself that his behavior was crazy and he needed to stop, but that logic could not penetrate into his damaged psyche, where the decisions were really coming from.

Thank God he called us that day and confessed everything. "I'm broken. I need help."

Teddy told us about a place he wanted to go for help, a facility called Warriors Heart. He couldn't afford it, so we called a man who'd been taking shooting lessons from Tom and who owned a large corporation and asked him if he would be willing to sponsor Teddy. This person wrote a blank check, which saved Teddy's life. Our friend went in for fourteen weeks, but he came out a completely different man. He's been clean and sober three years now, and he's on the Warriors Heart advisory board of directors. He has a new mission, a new purpose, a new life. He fully grasps how alcohol and drugs were fueling the raging wildfire that is PTSD. The only way to combat that enemy is to gather trained troops around you—to get professional help.

When Tom and I see him now, he is calm and a much deeper thinker than I'd given him credit for, entertaining us with interesting philosophical conversations versus breaking pool cues or slamming down a bottle of tequila. The amount of courage it took for him to ask for help, a person trained to be the savior, not the needy, is unfathomable. Teddy picked up that ten-thousand-pound phone and called us. The strength and resiliency he exerted is beyond admirable.

There are so many success stories, warriors who have completely turned around their lives, their jobs, their families, because they got sober. When they stopped drinking and doing drugs, they were then able to consciously go to battle with the other symptoms destroying their lives. A warrior wouldn't want a brother going into combat with him if he was wasted. Warriors need to be sharp and focused in a fight, lives are on the line. If your warrior is suffering from PTSD, it's important to remind them that this *is* a battle, and if they want to save themselves and those around them, they need to gather their courage, they need to have their wits about them, and they need to charge into the mission of healing, fully committed.

I'm going to talk about modes of healing later, but the first step is for those who are suffering to reach out to someone who is in a position to help. Talking to a friend about the problems is great and very healthy, but if your friend doesn't know anything about recovery programs, or PTSD, or have contacts with addiction or mental health professionals, then they are not the right person to rely on for anything beyond encouragement and caring. Get out your laptop and look up services in your area or for military support organizations. Our nonprofit, All Secure, keeps a list of updated references and contacts on the website, allsecurefoundation.org. Get a phone number for a specialist from a friend. Start with that call. If they can't help you, keep calling. Your mission has just started, don't lie down and give up now.

Infidelity

"He comes home late, climbs into bed, tells me in this boozy voice how much he loves me, begging me not to leave him, reeking of a different perfume every night. I can handle the drinking, usually, but this…"

A story I hear again and again. Affairs are nothing if not reckless.

There's a movie out there that 1.5 million of us have seen and loved, even with two main characters who are cheating cheaters. I'm talking, of course, about *The Notebook*. Sure, they're sweet, a spunky Southern girl with a good heart and a handsome boy from the wrong side of the tracks, but when they finally fall into bed together, she's engaged to someone else. It doesn't matter. We all cheer at the "happy" ending.

Hollywood has led us down this road many times, presenting love triangles in ways that we end up supporting the couples we adore, even if they've hurt other people. I mean, didn't you root for Harry and Sally to figure it out and get together when they were dating other people? Very rarely does a viewer turn on their beloved character, muttering, *Well, she's a bitch. She had an affair and she's going to burn in Hell.* Instead, we like love working out, so we withhold judgment.

Well, in fantasyland, anyway, or maybe in the surreal world of rock stars. But in the real world? Not so much. We are hard on the people in our lives who have affairs. Righteous. The Allie and Noahs of the fictional world are not treated the same as the Tom and Jens of the real world.

By revealing here that Tom and I came together when we were still with other partners, I know I will be judged. Harshly. Rightly so, maybe. I'm not proud of it. Yet, I'm also so, so grateful that I found this man, my Tom, both of us deeply lonely before we met. Those people outside of my circle making judgments are doing so only on a single action, not the big picture. Everybody's story is different. When I reveal that Tom had an emotional affair during the first year of our marriage, some will say, "God, what a weak woman for staying with a man like that. A strong woman would leave," ignoring how an even stronger woman or man, if they value their partnership and decide it is worth it to stay, will pull up the person who has fallen and figure out how to reconnect. For Tom, trying to control and overcome the disconnect he felt with me and the world around him was part of his PTSD.

So, why am I revealing this very personal, incredibly painful and embarrassing part of my past? Because, in order for me to talk about infidelity, I need to be as open as I'm going to ask you and your partner to be. Because infidelity in the military is rampant. High-risk behavior is a symptom of PTSD, and infidelity is definitely a risky thrill ride, which Tom and I learned the hard way. But we're going to help you to understand and to better control what's going on.

Don't get me wrong, I'm not saying anyone who has an affair is suffering from PTSD. Far from it. But the reasons for infidelity usually boil down to trying to find a fulfilling connection when you feel disconnected from the rest of your relationships, according to Dr. Sue Johnson. I believe that. People with PTSD are as disconnected as they come.

I really want to make sure you understand that when I start talking about the military guys and gals and affairs, I am not in any way saying they are worse, or better, than civilians. It's just that there's a stigma attached to the military community, thinking of them as bad boys or slutty girls, swaggering through the bars with macho bravado. It certainly is part of their culture, doing whatever is risky and dangerous, from driving too fast, to fights, to drinking, to hooking up, whatever it takes to make them feel alive and look good to their fellow adrenaline junkies.

The Disconnect

In the military community, bravado and reckless behavior is encouraged. I saw it all the time, every training exercise I went on. This is not to say that every Seal Team member was getting in fights or stepping out, but there were always a handful of married guys who were at the bars, hooking up with strangers, and then openly talking about it to the other guys. It was commonplace.

It's a scary thing for warrior wives, because we know this huge, ugly thing is out there. We know it happens. We know it's acceptable, or at least made to look that way. I don't want to create unnecessary anxiety or panic in the partners at home—I meet a lot of soldiers who adore their wives, who talk about their kids, who tell me they would never do that to their spouse. But even if your man is true to you, most of these loving family men are not stopping their married buddies from picking up women. They are not helping others to be better. Half the time, they are egging on their teammates, "Yeah, get you some of that, buddy." I've also seen firsthand how civilian women and men are attracted to our warriors; the choice of hooking up is dangled in front of the soldiers constantly.

Like I said, though, it doesn't mean your man or woman is part of the statistic! Talk to your partner, work with them, evaluate your connection. If you're at a good place, then it doesn't matter how many people advance on your spouse.

The sad reality about military life, though, is that disconnection is built into the system. If you have chosen to marry a person in the armed forces, then you have also made the choice to be in a relationship that is knowingly more challenging than most. Your spouse is going to deploy, they will be physically disconnected from you for months and months on end, and, eventually, emotionally disconnected. When they come home on leave, you have a short time to discover each other again, and then he's going to rotate back out. You can only hope that during the brief intermission, he is able to put aside the stress from the field long enough that he can let you in, and that you can do the same for him, managing your expectations while knowing you are with a person whose job it is to put the mission first. The longer the deployments, the amount of training exercises…it's wearing. It tears him down, it tears you down, and it can tear down the relationship.

If your partner is struggling with PTSD, then infidelity is even more of a concern. When they are home, often they want to reconnect with their families, but their mind won't let them switch over from warrior mode to cuddly husband mode, not easily. Remember, PTSD changes the biological functions in the brain, including inhibiting the person from feeling anything, especially joy or empathy. The more they spiral out of control, the more they disconnect from the family, oftentimes out of fear that they will hurt them, and/or because it feels like no one understands the crazy, mixed-up signals firing in their brain, or the inability to control the rages. As the depression and anger grow, the disconnect grows. As the warrior pushes away his wife, so, too, does she further the disconnect, barricading her heart against the abuse.

Most humans crave connection, so if they are failing at home, they try to fill that need wherever they can. Throw in the adrenaline rush of the chase and the thrill of possibly getting caught, then affairs are tailor-made for military personnel with PTSD, who do dangerous things just to feel alive.

So, it's not crazy that military people have affairs and divorces. It is said that about 50 percent of civilian partners cheat and, while there are various, contradictory statistics about military personnel, I'd say after hearing hundreds and hundreds of stories, it's higher. Also, I have never met civilian people who have been married four times, but that is far from rare in the military or with first responders. I mean, I'm Tom's fourth wife.

You will always have to be working toward staying connected. Air out problems when you have them. If you wait, conflicts turn into grudges. Find resolutions that both of you can agree to. Get counseling, even if things seem to be going well. If you want a happy relationship, you have to work for a happy relationship. Establish clear guidelines on what's acceptable in your marriage. You would think, well, that's a fucking no-brainer, right? Like, obviously, cheating is out. But what do you consider cheating? Be explicit. Sending flirty emails, or texting or calling using intimate language or photos…that is an affair. Even if you have not been physically intimate with someone, writing or verbally engaging with sexualized or intimate dialogue means you are engaging in a relationship with someone other than your spouse. An emotional affair is still cheating. Facebook and other social media platforms are blamed for a large number of divorces, because so many people are reaching out to old flings or meeting new people online; be clear with your partner that is not acceptable. Better yet, share accounts. Share computer passwords. If you don't have communication about what's acceptable to you and what's not, where the line is drawn for you, now is the time. Create a contract and both of you sign it.

Maybe an affair has already happened. What then?

How Do I Forgive?

I've told you, the first years of my relationship were in shambles, an emotional rollercoaster that I wanted to jump free from almost as often as I enjoyed the ride. We didn't understand the first thing about PTSD. Tom came into it believing that of course he didn't have a disorder, that he was no "weakling." For my part, I hadn't realized how many symptoms of PTSD I had been managing in myself, thanks to suppressing my childhood trauma and a rape, and I certainly hadn't known there was such a thing as secondary PTSD, caused by living on edge every second of every day, prepared to flee or do battle when my loving Jekyll inevitably turned into the violent Hyde.

By the time Tom was diagnosed and came to accept it, and I accepted my own truths, our disconnect was significant. We wanted to be in love, we wanted to be together, but there were so many walls between us. I had turned inward or toward friends. Tom, his insides too messy and chaotic to face, sought connection outside.

I can't count the number of times I've gotten the call, "Hey, my wife found out I had an affair and she wants to leave and take the kids. Can you call her? Please, can you help me get her back?"

When I ask why the affair happened in the first place, it's most often because of a deployment and then an inability to get on the same page again once they are back home. Often, the warrior can't see how their behavior, which worked for them when they were away, was causing discord at home. The self-isolating, the lashing out, going out with the guys every night, not helping out around home, treating their partner like a bro—or worse—like an enemy, instead of with love and respect…the partner inevitably shuts themselves off, protects themselves, just like the soldier has, though both at their core really only want to be loved. Both parties feel alone, angry, and bitter. The door has been opened for someone else to walk in, to fill the void. In those moments of vulnerability, especially if the mind is clouded by alcohol and depression, an affair can happen.

Few things unravel a relationship faster than infidelity.

Facing down your warrior's demons is uncomfortable, sometimes dangerous—it's easier to fight about unfinished laundry than to get into it over amoral behavior. The surface issues are hard enough to deal with, but they will only continue to escalate unless the underscoring issue, the PTSD, is addressed. Many military couples end up avoiding each other altogether because the interactions between them have become so unpleasant and often damaging. The relationship starts to crack. When affairs are discovered, the distance between you can seem insurmountable.

First, establish that you both want to save the relationship. Then, it is time to step out of your egos and consider the relationship as a third party. With us, there is Tom, there is Jen, and there is Us. Our old pattern was for me to put myself first, and Tom to put himself first, which meant our relationship was last. Both Tom and I wanted to stay together, so we had to make the promise that, before we said anything or made decisions or reacted, we would pause and consciously process these questions: Is this good for *us* or is this good for *me*? If the answer was that it was good for me, then I would ask myself: It might be good for me, but is it bad for Us? If so, then it was time to reevaluate how to proceed.

That all sounds very logical, doesn't it? But I'm sure it's the emotional side you want to know about. How can you forgive the cheater?

Here's how I did it, though I have to admit I didn't find out about the affair until years after the fact, which changed how I would have digested the information. Luckily for us, I had spent those first years of our marriage watching Tom become a better, stronger human, diligently working his way through six or seven different healing modalities. We walked through every one of those modalities together. Every Transcendental Meditation appointment, I was there, every therapy appointment. I was there doing research and ordering of all of his supplements. I was at every appointment that he had for doctors or chiropractors or pain management. I went when he started TMS, transcranial magnetic stimulation. When he got his brain zapped five days a week for eight weeks. I went to every single appointment to combat PTSD for over three years—and I saw him change. When some of the PTSD shit started to wash away, then I saw the real Tom more and more.

So, three years into the marriage, when I found out about Tom and a long-term flirtation with a retired Army woman he met while contracting when we were first married, I was rocked to my core, blown apart...but I really heard Tom when he said, "Wait! I'm not that man anymore."

He was right. How could I judge him for a mistake made before he understood his condition? How could I leave him when I had made the same mistake, falling for Tom before I was divorced from my first husband?

Besides, the disconnect between us back then had been unbearable. Our first year married felt like ten. We had gone through so many challenges and struggles, and we were both wounded. I would repeatedly tell Tom, "You're drinking too much. You're angry too much." It was true and coming out of a place of love and concern, but the way I went about constantly telling him how broken he was didn't help. I was leaving the door open for somebody to make him feel good about himself and he took it, and I can't shame him about it for the rest of his life.

Back then, there was a hole needing to be filled. I dove into health coaching school and became very close to a couple of women in that community; they filled some of the void for me. We had a friendship. We talked every day. I felt connected.

Tom was in a bad place, alone and feeling judged. His PTSD was raging. He was working with a woman who became very attentive. The thrill of the risk of an affair outweighed the harms of losing his new marriage. It was his habit to go forward with reckless abandon, the same "fuck it" attitude he had when re-pelling off buildings, dropping ninety feet on fast rope from a helicopter, or doing HALO jumps from thirty thousand feet, or surviving massive battles where he should have died, finding bullet holes in his clothing after a combat mission. When you feel like you're going to die and then you don't, you develop a very strange, God-like way of thinking: *I made it through. There are no consequences.* And, so, the behavior becomes riskier and riskier, needing a bigger rush of adrenaline.

Tom admitted he had flirted with women at the bars back then, but the woman he worked alongside was a prolonged inter-action. At first, it was friendly banter, and then texting, and then flirty texting. For months, he was having these long, personal, and sometimes sexualized conversations with the woman.

I knew the emotional affair was just one piece in what had been a broken marriage at the time. We'd mended so many of the other pieces, was I going to throw away this beautiful thing we had going because of past mistakes? I was given the luxury of time before finding out about it, to see that neither of us were the same people we had been at the time.

I don't ask for apologies anymore. That's done. If your partner has sincerely apologized and has every intention of staying faithful, then you have to stop bringing it up in a pejorative manner. Let that wound scar up, start to heal.

Tom was completely open and willing to hear my pain. I hope other warriors and warrior spouses who have cheated will allow for that, because it was very healing for me. And I mean, I got it out for days on end. And I know how every time I talked about it, it put him into a shame spiral. Yet, he let me talk about it. He encouraged me. He held me when I cried. I would have a fit, and he was of the mindset that he deserved it, saying, "Whatever you need to do to heal. Whatever you need."

Tom was heartbroken that he'd hurt me and he'd hurt Us. It crushed him to see me sobbing because of something he'd done. The pain was there for the both of us. Instead of avoiding it or playing games, we just held it, let it be, saw and accepted it. The source of the pain was sorrow, which had become a boulder that was crushing Us. But just like that guy who sawed off his own arm to escape from a boulder, I was willing to do what it took to get that boulder off of Us.

I never once told Tom I was going to leave him. In fact, he would ask all the time, "Are you going to leave?" And my answer was always, "No, we'll get through this. This is another challenge. This is just another shitstorm and we will be stronger when we get to the other side."

Two weeks after I found out about it, a friend asked me, "How are you able to forgive Tom so quickly? I can't believe how well you're doing. You seem totally fine."

I said, "I'm not totally fine. I'm still unbelievably hurt. I'm processing it, but that pain doesn't define me. I'm going to deal with it the best I can."

We individually started seeing Stacey, the therapist, but more frequently as a couple. I would not let it destroy Us. There'll be a part of me that will always hurt that he turned to another woman, but it won't define our relationship now. It won't make or break Us. It's part of our path that we've traveled together. It's part of our experience as a couple.

If you got an Us worth fighting for, fight for it. I said my wedding vows, for good times and bad. There's been a lot of bad. There's also been a tremendous amount of good—and I am not willing to get rid of our great, fucking phenomenal good. But the reckless behavior has gotta go.

FIVE

The Grinch who Steals Christmas—and Birthdays: Survivor's Guilt and Moral Injury

On the day after Christmas, I received a text message early in the morning. It was from a warrior spouse I had spoken with a few weeks prior, a woman who told me how her Special Forces husband had PTSD and the symptoms were steadily getting worse. Sadly, it wasn't a huge surprise to get a plea for help on December 26.

In fact, she was one of three military spouses who reached out to me that day.

Holidays are stressful for the calmest of people, but the abandoned routines and surprise visitors and last-minute holiday duties and everyone else's stress are a type of chaos that is difficult to assimilate for someone with PTSD.

To make matters worse, most combat veterans struggle during the holidays, acknowledging they are alive and with family while so many of their brothers and sisters in arms are no longer with us, having died thousands of miles from their loved ones. This is survivor's guilt, common with military or first responders who have complex PTSD.

I steeled myself for an emotional conversation and called the wife. She picked up but then couldn't utter a word for ten minutes. Instead, she gasped and broke into sobs. I told her to let it out and to take as long as she needed. She'd get herself calm, start to talk, and then sob, then start, and then sob. I told her to relax and take some deep breaths, I wasn't going anywhere, so she cried it out for a few more minutes. Finally, she was able to verbalize the pain she was holding in her heart.

She told me about how she had saved for months in order to buy nice Christmas presents for their young children and had been cooking and cleaning for a week, getting ready for the holiday. Christmas day, she woke up early and made a special breakfast and decorated the house with love. She was looking forward to a great morning, like the ones on Facebook, where everyone is smiling and laughing and opening presents and eventually passed out by the fire after a huge dinner. But she was also cautious, not knowing the mood her husband would be in. Holidays were often a trigger for Mike.

"I want my kids to remember Christmas as a happy time," she told me. "To create memories to be built on, when they are grown with their own children. I want them to remember Christmas mornings as something special…" She broke down again. When she was able to continue, her voice was shaky and quiet. To have this conversation, she'd hidden in her bathroom, not wanting the kids to hear her sadness, her hurt. The pain of another ruined holiday had affected her children, and she didn't know what to do or who to turn to.

"He spent the entire morning in bed. When he finally came out, he immediately started barking orders at me and the kids, becoming angrier and angrier, and ended up leaving for a few hours. The day was totally ruined. Will I ever have a normal Christmas again?"

Like so many other warrior spouses, she felt completely alone in this struggle.

I told her she had me, she wasn't alone, and that, in fact, I hadn't had a holiday without some sort of issue or struggle in seven years.

Active duty spouses tend to have no idea that the house next door to them on the base is going through the same thing, and the same is true five doors down, seven doors down, and so on. No, not every soldier has PTSD, not even close, and also not every soldier with PTSD has issues with celebration, but many, many do. How many? It's too hard to say, it's not something that families advertise: "Dear world, my spouse really fucks up every holiday, every birthday, and every celebration. It makes him feel like a massive asshole later and I know he truly hates himself for it, but now our kids are traumatized."

So, yes, I get it.

I can't "fix" a relationship or make a Christmas great for others, but I can arm families with knowledge about what's happening and why it's happening, and I can give a compass for them to use to navigate their way out of the forest.

Manage Your Expectations, Clark Griswold

Ruined holidays and celebrations were no stranger to us. Just about every birthday, holiday, or special event since we met had a dark cloud over it—or full-on tornado. The first time I saw this unfold in our relationship was on my fortieth birthday, a few months after we married. I thought a small gathering with a few of my closest friends was exactly the kind of night I wanted to welcome in a new decade. Unfortunately, the planning process became overly complicated. Every time I tried to work out the details, Tom seemed agitated; I kept assuring him that he wouldn't have to do anything, just show up. I thought by "letting him off the hook," not asking him to clean, shop, cook, decorate, or really anything, that he'd be stress-free. He'd be fine.

Yet, because he has a deep-seated need to be in control, he insisted on helping. Unfortunately, he'd give himself some task and then spend the entire time complaining bitterly.

His complaints never had anything to do with my friends, but with me. He always came back a few hours later with a murmur of an apology, though somehow always turned it back on me and how I was at fault for his childish behavior or backhanded comments. I told him that his way of apologizing sucked. It was never, "I'm sorry." It was, "I'm sorry, but…"

Back then, to him, apologizing meant admitting fault, which was admitting weakness. I'd seen him take responsibility for errors in work situations with no problem, even if they weren't his, but in an intimate relationship, things were much different.

Tom was being rude, sometimes mean. Inevitably, the party became this heavy thing that I was dreading. The joy had been sucked out of it. But I was too embarrassed to cancel. I didn't want to say, "You guys can't come over, my husband is being a royal dick."

The party came and everyone had a great time. Tom included. He was relaxed, funny, and helped in every way. It was a great night. I was relieved but couldn't understand why he'd offered me so much anger and resentment beforehand.

During that first year of marriage, planning for holidays, anniversaries, weddings, and birthdays was all met with the same anger and confused frustration. I asked Tom many times why happy occasions made him so upset. We had yet to learn how his subconscious was still stuck in battle mode. Back then, he was unable to put a finger on what was happening to him.

"I don't know, Jen. I think it's because I see everyone gathered and happy and then something goes wrong, like the kids bickering at each other, or the dog eating the donuts, or how the ideal holiday I created in my mind never plays out as I pictured. Once something goes wrong, no matter how small, then I feel like...fuck it, it's all ruined. I have these huge expectations for perfection. I know it's not logical, but that's where my head goes."

Once Tom started to approach holidays or vacations with lower expectations and planned for less than perfect, he was more at peace. This last vacation to the Smoky Mountains was our best vacation to date, seven years after we met. He took it as a time to get away with the kids, deliberately leaving his expectations at home. He was happier than I've ever seen him on a trip. Things weren't perfect, because life isn't perfect, and there was a small outburst on day five…but most couples argue at some point on a vacation, right? You need to look at your life like some of this stuff is just normal. PTSD isn't always at play. If you're tired, hungry, and the kids are punching each other in the backseat, every parent in America is eventually going to whip around and threaten the kids with being left by the side of the road. Everyone pops from time to time.

On top of this, Tom struggled to define his guilt. "My friends are dead, their families without them, yet here I sit with my family. Everything is going normally here, like nothing has happened. But I'm here and they're not. I feel so ashamed that I can be with my family and they will never be whole again, not like us. How can everyone be so happy with so much bullshit in the world?"

Jealousy also plays a role in survivor's guilt but, again, not at a conscious level. Tom had been left here to deal with reality. The chaos and the ugliness. He no longer was able to experience moments of pure, unobstructed joy. "I wish I could be like you guys, so happy and free, without any memories of really bad things. I envy your purity. I remember what it was like before, when I was a kid, but I don't feel I can ever have that kind of happiness again; when I see you being happy, I want it and sometimes it makes me jealous, bitter. Then I feel ashamed and guilty for begrudging your happiness."

Acknowledging the Source...and the Response

October third has always been a tough date. This was the day twenty-seven years ago that changed Tom forever. The Battle of Mogadishu, the basis for the movie *Black Hawk Down*. Tom was part of the infamous street battle, the longest sustained firefight since Vietnam. Surrounded by thousands of militia wanting nothing more than to kill him, an elite American soldier, the twenty-six-year old faced down what he believed was the last night of his life. Up until then, Tom had believed himself invincible, like he could do anything and his training would keep him and his brothers alive. The harsh, deadly reality of mortality in war came crashing in when the walls of a small, two-room house where they were taking refuge blew in around them. He lost nineteen brothers within seventeen hours, and his heart and mind were never the same.

Each anniversary of the battle, Tom found his way into a bar, attempting to drink away the memories. After years of this, his depression had only become blacker and more debilitating. It took years of work to get him to acknowledge the guilt he carried over surviving while his brothers died, as well as his harmful responses to that guilt.

On October 3, 2016, instead of spending time in bars, he was with me, at my daughter's ninth birthday party. We had family over and it wasn't until the end of the day, when he reminded me, that I remembered what day it was. I felt terrible, but then it hit me...he'd actually had a great day, talking, laughing, and helping out. When we put our feet up at the end that evening, we talked about it. He told me it was the first year that he hadn't felt the need to drink the memories and feelings away.

I had certainly never blamed him for doing so, not when there was so much pain, so much loss, so much fear. It was no wonder he wanted to drink it away.

After a long pause, I asked, "How would Gary, Randy, Earl, Tim, Matt, and Dan, and the Ranger soldiers who were killed that day want to see you? In despair and drinking out the entire bar? Or would they rather see you surrounded by family, happy and enjoying your life? What would you want for them if it was reversed?"

He sat with that for a while. "They would want me to be happy, and I would want that for them, too."

Did that light bulb moment completely erase his survivor's guilt? No, but it helped. And every bit of movement toward the light is a good move.

There were still bad times, to be sure.

So, over the years, I would come up with game plans for handling Tom as we approached the holidays. Tom, understandably, didn't appreciate being handled like a child, but I would sometimes unintentionally act like a mama bear instead of a partner. I was trying to protect him as much as everyone else in our family, wanting everyone to experience joy on the holidays.

Leading up to the events, I would prepare him with my expectations. Never over the top, pie-in-the-sky requests, just, "Hey, can you show a happy face on Christmas? I really want you to enjoy it. What can I do to help you have a good day?"

These requests, no matter how carefully stated, only managed to set off his guilt, reinforcing how many days he'd ruined for us in the past. He didn't yet know how to process it, which then just made him angry. "I don't need you to tell me to have a good Christmas! I'm not a fucking child, I can handle it. I won't fucking ruin it for you or the kids, okay?"

Watching him walk off in a huff, I asked myself how I could do it differently. I kept thinking if I talked to him about it beforehand that it would help, but it rarely did. So, then I would try to ignore the elephant in the room and just make very passive comments about the upcoming holiday. Every comment I made, no matter how light, was treated as if I was browbeating him.

Finally, I would just ignore the upcoming date entirely if he was around, like if I didn't acknowledge it, maybe life would proceed normally, no fuss. Yeah. That definitely didn't work, either.

This year, we came into the holidays with a much better understanding of PTSD, Tom's triggers, and some methods for helping him manage them.

My kids, now teenagers, spent Christmas Eve at their father's house, leaving Tom and I to wake up to a quiet Christmas morning. Tom was able to ease into the day. By the time the kids were dropped off at noon, the holiday lunch was on the table and presents by the tree, and everything felt calm and under control. Tom was prepared. He said he didn't care if the kids tore into presents and left a mess, he didn't care if the kids got into an argument, knowing that's what teens did. He told himself he didn't care if lunch or dinner wasn't perfect. He'd lowered his expectations and removed the pressure. It worked. It was our best holiday to date. I felt like the nut had been cracked. Maybe we wouldn't have to deal with the Grinch anymore.

Fast forward a few months to Easter. He woke up grumpy, though he'd been fine the night before. He isolated most of the day in his room, watching TV. When he did surface, he was distant and cold, keeping himself sequestered instead of taking out his angst on us. I left him alone and went on with my day, knowing not to push. We managed our emotions. It didn't make for a perfect day, or even a satisfactory day, but we made it through.

That's the hardest thing about PTSD: ten steps forward, five back. But that's really true for most of us; we all move forward, and we all have setbacks. Understanding that has kept me sane.

Another thing I have come to understand is that the wounds and the treatments are not black and white. These soldiers have been walking through a gray world, the ground below them always shifting, as they make constant life-and-death decisions. Then they come home and feel guilty for being in a safe environment with loved ones when others did not make it. Going hand-in-hand with that is also the guilt over who they've become.

And what they have done.

Moral Injury

During my time embedded with Special Operations, I've talked to soldiers about a myriad of topics, from war, to barbecue recipes and making your own beer, to raising kids.

One of the guys I worked with during the trainings was literally a genius, having studied quantum physics, and we once talked for several hours about the existence of God from a scientific viewpoint. I was so fascinated by his big, complex theories that I ended up going home and buying books about the topic.

But very few guys in the field would get together and talk about religion or God. It wasn't until I began working one-on-one with soldiers that I began to hear their more existential struggles. Most of the time, it would begin with them just talking, me letting them tell their stories—they didn't want to burden their wives or families with the ugly parts of war, but I was someone unrelated, almost anonymous.

I would hear some of their deepest, darkest secrets or thoughts, most of which would make me cry and rage for them. Some would make me laugh my ass off. I swear, the funniest people I have met work in Special Operations. Smartass is part of the culture in a big way. But humor is just one more coping mechanism, using it to stave off the ugliness trying to take over.

Some of their secrets would rattle me to my core. For them, the result of holding onto their secrets and dark stories was sometimes devastating.

"It doesn't matter what I do now. Why should it? I'm going to Hell anyway."

The young Ranger on the other end of the phone was twenty-eight and lost in despair. I couldn't imagine thinking my life was completely hopeless and not worth living by the age of twenty-eight.

"Do you really believe that? You've been serving our country. Do you really think you're going to Hell when you were doing what you were ordered to do, to protect us?"

"Absolutely," he said without hesitation. "Which means, what's the point of going on? Or, if I do stick around, what's the point of living any kind of good life? I'm going to Hell no matter what choices I make now."

The Ranger told me he was from a small town in Kentucky, raised in the Southern Baptist church. He'd been taught from the day he was born until the day he enlisted that killing was wrong. Hurting people was wrong.

Do unto others as you'd have done unto you, it said in the Bible. It was in the Commandments that thou shalt not murder. His kindergarten teacher drilled into him, "Do not hurt others. It is wrong to do so." The church would tell him it was a sin.

This Ranger had been forced to abandon what he knew as "right" and "good" in order to do what the government asked of him overseas. For the greater good, he gave up who he knew himself to be, a decent and moral person, and became what he needed to be. A warrior trained to kill when deemed necessary. He gave up his "eligibility for Heaven."

Now, he couldn't bear to look his parents in the eye, so he just didn't go home.

"Don't you think your parents love you no matter what? Unconditionally? Aren't they proud of you and your service to this country? I'm sure they are. I'm sure they miss you terribly and they're very worried about you."

He couldn't or wouldn't hear it. He had a mental list of the terrible things he'd done to others in the name of democracy, and had made up his mind that his parents would judge him, his town would judge him, and he was already judging himself enough.

"If they knew the shit that I had to do, I don't think they would love me anymore. I mean, I think they might *love* me, but not in the same way. I know they wouldn't look at me the same.

I don't want my mom to know those things about me, I don't want her to look at me any differently. I couldn't handle that."

His sense of morality, a core tenant of how he defined himself, had been traumatized. Hence, the term "moral injury," which was coined by a psychiatrist in the 1990s, though this type of anguish over perceived moral transgressions has been called different things over the centuries. Since the start of wars, soldiers have gone into battle and, if lucky enough, stumbled home alive, but often dealing with an overwhelming shame because they had killed another human being and anger because those whom they had been protecting considered the acts required of the soldier to be reprehensible.

Rev. Dr. Gabriella Lettini, a professor of theological ethics, defines moral injury not as a psychological disorder, but as "souls in anguish." On the Brite Divinity School website (https://brite. edu/programs/soul-repair), Rev. Dr. Lettini states, "This occurs when veterans struggle with a lost sense of humanity after transgressing deeply held moral beliefs."

I believe that to be true. Over the years, I've had many conversations with soldiers who have made comments similar to the young Ranger, claiming that although it had been their duty to take a human life, trained by the military to be effective at taking out the "enemy," they couldn't make peace with what they'd done. They'd grown up believing killing to be wrong, even evil, no matter the reason. It only made matters worse that they spent their time overseas hurting others only to return home very deeply changed. "I'm a monster," I heard more than once. They could see themselves still acting like soldiers in battle, being aggressive, angry, and even sometimes abusive to those they loved, but they felt out of control to stop it.

The absolute worst was when they'd realize they were justifying their terrible behavior or actions and yet no longer cared. They believed they'd become evil and were beyond redemption, broken creatures.

Getting to This Place

When I first started working in Special Operations, it was really disturbing to me to see soldiers cheering at a death while watching footage of skirmishes, or just the way that annihilating an "enemy" could be turned into a form of comedy.

"Did you see the way that fucker's head blew up?"

"BOOM! Those assholes are like sausages on a grill. Burnt up and then gone!"

While I hadn't been in combat, I had seen my share of "Kill TV," as Tom called it—the ISR footage of missions, captures, and kills. It doesn't look like much on the little black-and-white screens in the viewing rooms, and most of the shots are from far away, but the way the men would watch and laugh and make fun of death bothered me.

"Tom, why do you guys do that?"

"We have to," he said. "We have to dehumanize the enemy. It's the only way we can do what we need to do. We are trained to kill because we have to kill. After time, you just end up dehumanizing everybody, including, I guess, sometimes myself and my family..."

He'd obviously thought of it before, the way his face turned red.

"Is it a conscious thought for you? About the lives you've taken? About what it means for you and your family?"

"No," he said. "That's how we're trained to think."

When I first met him and we had these conversations, he would become agitated, angry, and defensive. "I hate when people ask me how many people I fucking killed. I don't know how many fucking people I've killed. I know it's a lot. And I know they all fucking deserved it. Every single one of them. I don't regret taking a single life, not for a minute."

I never asked him how many people he killed, though he has been asked that before, many times. I also never meant to bring judgment with the questions I did ask, but now I can see that I did judge him, and I only deepened his guilt. It was unintentional, it was thoughtless. My questions came from a place of curiosity, my anthropology background coming to the forefront, but it was still callous on many levels. I'd felt that I had to understand in order to help in some way.

It boils down to the fact that taking human lives is a part of being in Special Forces. Dealing with the aftermath is also a big part of it. There is no healing without it. But to admit that the enemy is human is to admit taking a human life.

I remember reading something in high school, something we were studying about World War II, the journal of a supposed enemy, a German soldier. It broke my heart in half. This young boy of nineteen or twenty years old talked about missing his mom and dad, missing his sister, missing his small town, missing his life. He talked about doing his duty, although he had issues with killing. He had issues with all of it. At the end of the essay, that German soldier died. He was buried in his small town and that was it.

We students were meant to think about people as people, the opposite of dehumanizing. I never forgot that story, about a young boy who missed his parents, who missed his hometown and the comfort of his bed and the foods he loved, fighting a war he didn't want to fight, killing people he didn't want to kill—just like any of our American boys.

I told Tom about this assignment.

"Of course. They are somebody's son or daughter, and they are taught what they are taught, just like we are taught what we are taught. We are all fighting against someone else's ideals, we are fighting against someone else's religion, we are fighting against politicians…we aren't fighting the soldier."

Given time to think and move away from conditioned response, he no longer found it exhilarating when we watched enemy combatants get killed. He came back to who he was.

It took Tom some time to get there, though, to see that it did actually bother him to take a human life. For years, he was the definition of macho, the tough American soldier who celebrated his kills. Not in an arrogant, flashy way, mind you. Tom was never that guy. I knew plenty of those guys, but Tom wasn't one of them. He was always quiet. He was always professional. He was an elite weapon, honed by the American military. But, in the end, he was also a human, like the rest of us.

The Answer

In an article by Dr. Camille Gaudet and associates entitled "A Review of PTSD and Shame in Military Veterans," published in the *Journal of Human Behavior in the Social Environment*, the lack of treatment in moral injury is obvious, and many health care providers are treating a complex moral injury as if they are treating depression. New treatment interventions need to be developed.

Working with people who suffer from PTSD has sometimes made me think I have to have all of the answers, but that's just not realistic. I have talked to seasoned doctors and therapists; I have interviewed soldiers, spouses, first responders, crime victims, researchers, and spiritual gurus; gathering dozens of different responses; and I have come to find there is no one solution, and certainly no easy solution. I wish I had more concrete answers on how to constructively handle many of the elements of PTSD—but I do feel pretty solid about the advice I'm about to give on moral injury.

Some believe that by combating the underlying issue of growing shame surrounding the moral injury, a tortured soul can be "repaired." Tom and I have come to see the truth in what some researchers are saying in this regard: service to others is the best medicine.

Remember when your mama or your grandma would tell you, "Do unto others as you'd have done unto you"? That golden rule isn't in place just to keep us in check when we are about to do something bad...it's also a reminder that we need to reach out to those who are suffering or who are in need. And when we do, the resulting good "feeling" is an actual physical response, as oxytocin, endorphins, and dopamine are released in your body. Your brain is rewarding you with pleasure.

You might argue then you're really doing the good deed for yourself, making it actually a selfish act, not altruistic. That kind of thinking is self-defeating and doesn't get us anywhere. Besides, if you've already served in the military, why stop serving now? We need to make sure we are helping out in our community, keeping our people strong and safe, and if making others feel warm and fuzzy makes *you* feel warm and fuzzy, all the better.

We are developing a new program at All Secure Foundation called Never Stop Serving, where we encourage those suffering to focus their energy on others in need, helping them find a volunteer opportunity that is a good fit. Recently, in a conversation with Sebastian Junger, extraordinary *NY Times* bestselling author of *Tribe: On Homecoming and Belonging* (and *The Perfect Storm*), I asked what he thought was most beneficial for PTSD recovery; he said it was for them to share their story. I agreed, telling him about Tom using his story to help others and how it also helped him. Then I told him about Never Stop Serving, and he said that consciously taking care of others would come in a close second.

This choice to serve started years ago, not long after I met Tom. He got a DUI and was completely mortified, but it was a wake-up call. That was when he first had to go to a therapist for anger management; he volunteered to keep going back when it was discovered he had complex PTSD.

He also was required to do community service. He put it off until the last minute. Finally, going over the list he'd been given of places where he could volunteer, we talked about it. He decided on a soup kitchen because he could get the hours done in the morning and get on with his day. He would have to go two and a half weeks, every morning, in order to fulfill his court order. There was so much nervousness and so much hesitation, I honestly thought he wouldn't go through with it.

"How was it?" I asked anxiously, when he called that first afternoon.

Driving away from the church annex, he told me he wasn't in love with the whole experience, but he didn't hate it, either. He wasn't surprised to learn that a few of the other guys were convicts from a halfway house. One guy, who was larger than life, stood out in particular because he was full of happiness. This left Tom conflicted—Raul didn't fit the mold of Tom's previous view on convicts.

Throughout the day, he'd served the men, women, and children, even calmly escorting out a man who was in a drunken rage. The director appreciated his efforts, which made him feel good. He enjoyed feeling useful.

After he'd served all his hours, Tom stayed on at the shelter for a few more weeks, until he moved to Savannah. He was helping others, he was having fun, he was breaking previous beliefs he held about homeless and convicts. He felt he belonged in this tribe of helpers he was working with. Giving back made him feel like he mattered again, like his life was worth something.

I knew exactly what he meant. I've spent a life in service, maybe in part to heal my own pain. I volunteered when I was twelve at a nursing home, then the hospital at fourteen, and various organizations through high school and college. It wasn't until my trip to the Dominican Republic with the Pujols Family Foundation that I knew my place was in serving others. I was the documentarian on a medical mission trip to some of the poorest parts of the DR, where famed all-star Albert Pujols grew up. And as a side note, this iconic baseball player said his favorite thing in the world was giving back; it sat below God and his family, but above baseball.

There is something to giving of yourself to others, the way it makes you feel, the lessons you learn, the people you meet, the sense of belonging to a tribe working together for good, the feeling of accomplishment when those you help are helped. It's beyond rewarding, it is life giving. As Winston Churchill famously stated, "We make a living by what we get. We make a life by what we give."

There is so much benefit to being part of something bigger than yourself that many organizations now are including service as part of healing. In fact, an Ivy League school has implemented service as part of depression healing. Students on campus who are depressed are encouraged to do service work, but it has to be out in the community, not with other college kids on campus. And it has worked; depression in those students went away, or at least they were doing so well that they didn't need college services anymore.

It's just as important for veterans to get out into their community, if not more so, to be reminded that they are not the only ones in need. They can use the many skills they've been taught in their time in the military to help others. Americans at home still need the warrior's help, just as he or she helped them by going overseas.

If you're in a relationship and think this might be of interest to you, volunteer as a couple or a family, double down on the good vibes. Tom and I always get a rush when we go out and give back together, we bond over it, we laugh and cry over it, we are stronger because of it. You don't have to go to Africa or South America, although I know a few families who have done both. Look to your neighborhood or community; start with the libraries, schools, homeless shelters, soup kitchens, fire departments, recreation centers, park cleanup or habitation programs, retirement homes, hospitals, or detention centers. Give back and, I promise you, if you find the right fit for your passion, you'll feel better.

SIX

Women Warriors Unite: When Spouses Isolate Themselves

MILITARY FAMILIES DON'T AIR DIRTY LAUNDRY. WE DON'T share the hurtful things, and definitely not the shameful. We want to create the image of the happy family. We desperately want to *be* an actual happy family. Yet, in a community of people with so many individuals silently suffering, it is surprising that most remain largely unaware that the person next door, and five doors down, and across the street, are going through the same tough times.

Tom explained it like this: "When you told your friends that you and Mark were getting divorced, remember what you found out? That nearly all of your friends, including some of your best friends, were going through or had gone through some serious relationship issues. In fact, one of your closest friends revealed that she had an affair, and another friend revealed she'd nearly got divorced a few years back, but you had no idea, and you consider them your best friends."

We hide what we can't face, or we hide what we're embarrassed about. Or we feel others don't need to know every last detail about what happens behind our closed doors. Why? Because we don't think others will understand.

How can they? Spouses don't even understand the changes in their partner. They *logically* know that their warrior has gone off and seen combat and will have endured horrific things, but when their warrior returns from deployment someone so different and less loving than the one who left, it just feels…incomprehensible. According to biopsychosocial health scientist Dr. Christi Luby, in a report called "Health Assessment for Loved Ones" (2015, University of Texas at El Paso), "Some spouse participants reported feeling distress due to the lack of understanding of changes in a Service member's behaviors and personality […]. Spouses noticed these changes before other close social or professional contacts recognized the differences […]. The military spouse and the children often tried to adapt to this new environment by changing how they reacted within the home and responded to the Service member."

Instead of reaching out for help, or even acknowledging something is wrong, we military spouses oftentimes play it off by "simply" adjusting our home life to meet the needs of our loved one. Even if those needs are irrational and, in the end, can never be met.

We engage in social avoidance because others won't understand...but maybe even more so because we don't want to be judged.

Marriage Shouldn't Be So Hard

Sure, you've thought it to yourself plenty of times, that marriage shouldn't be so goddamn hard...but it's totally different when your cousin or a friend listens to your stories, then sniffs and says righteously, "Geez, Jen, marriage isn't supposed to be so hard."

WTF?! How dare they! They don't know him. Obviously, they don't really know me. And they don't understand Us.

Then I realized...why should I have to justify my relationship to anyone else? If I tried to explain or rationalize our sometimes-crazy interactions, would it even make sense?

It didn't need to make sense for anyone else but me and him. So, I told myself to stop caring.

First, I stopped reading the "10 Reasons You Should Leave Him" and "How to Spot a Toxic Relationship" Facebook lists and blogs. *Because, honey, we were getting a 10 out of 10, and not in a good way.* Yet, that wasn't fair. We were good together. We simply didn't meet the conventional standards of some twenty-five-year old writer fresh out of school, in a new job in the big city. *Uh-huh. I'm glad the writer hasn't had the experience of loving someone with a past so dark, so trauma filled, so intense. I'm glad she's engaged to an accountant. Or a lawyer. Or a whatever. Maybe she doesn't even have a boyfriend.*

I stopped reading things that made me feel ashamed or embarrassed. I was tired of believing I should be the strong, independent woman who gets a 0 out of 10 on *Cosmo's* toxic relationship scale. I was pulling my hair out, thinking, *What would my strong female role models think about me being in a toxic relationship?*

In the end, it was easy to avoid stupid articles or relationship quizzes, but avoiding my parents or our friends was a whole other issue. I'd like to tell you that I didn't fear judgment. But I did.

I hadn't yet embraced the old Latin term *virago*, made it my own.

Virago: a woman of strength and spirit; a female warrior.

Choosing Social Isolation

During those first couple of years of marriage, I started avoiding going out. I didn't have bruises to hide, but it was not rare for me to have a puffy face from crying. I was often an emotional wreck, sometimes short with people, sometimes close to tears, rarely for a good reason. My natural easygoing personality felt like it had up and left, and now I was just an unhappy meat sack.

I did a good job of hiding it, mostly, from family and friends. I'd had a lot of practice, having spent years creating and wearing masks to hide pain or shame, and now was no different. I opened up with one or two very close friends but never to my family or other friends, who I thought would judge or ridicule my choice in partner. There were enough times I did that myself; I didn't need a cheering, or booing, section.

If Tom was around, it would be worse, as I was afraid he was going to switch from the charmer to the asshole at any second.

Dr. Luby's report, mentioned above, discusses this as well, that interviewed military spouses found certain forms of social interaction physically and emotionally exhausting, that they felt "they must be on guard and looking out for things that might trigger issues in their Service member when out in public or social settings."

Knowing I was worried about that, Tom resented it, obviously. I knew a meltdown or even sharp words with an angry overtone wouldn't fly around my family. They did not take discord lightly. Nor did they have any idea how bad Tom's PTSD was, and that the world was full of triggers he couldn't avoid, no matter how hard he tried.

Despite my desire to not justify myself to anyone, I did want to have a relationship with the other people in my life. I just couldn't talk about life at home.

How do I explain Us? How do I defend Us?

How do I defend him?

If I told them the real stories, the dark moments, my friends wouldn't understand and they'd tell me to leave him. My family definitely wouldn't understand—they'd push me to leave him.

I tried to explain the biological nature of PTSD and the behaviors and responses it can cause. Our family and friends usually said they understood, and they really wanted to, but unless you've seen the despair in Tom's eyes when he realizes Crawler has snapped into control, it's hard to conceptualize. Most people, their gut reaction is, "Come on, he didn't have to act that way. He's a grown man."

I want to make it clear that isolating yourself and shielding the person suffering from PTSD is not simply making your life complicated and unhappy. It can also be dangerous. PTSD only gets worse over time if left untreated, not better. Things in your house will not improve if you ignore it. The irrational behavior and responses will only increase and grow in intensity. Hiding the arguments and the broken furniture from the neighbors might protect your ego in the short term, but it will do permanent damage to everyone's psyche in the household if it continues, unacknowledged and unhindered. Inevitably, someone's going to get hurt, no matter how much love there is between you. PTSD is a beast, making the decisions in your house, if you let it.

Most people around us had no idea how hard Tom has had to fight in order to rewire the biology of his warrior-trained brain. *God, please fix him,* I'd pray. *Please make him okay. Please heal him. Please make this stop. I just want us to be normal.*

Full stop.

Did I just pray for normalcy?!

Never had I wanted a normal life. Never did I want the run-of-the-mill type of lifestyle. I wanted adventure. I wanted challenges. I wanted to be a badass.

Maybe my prayers had already been answered. Disguised, but answered.

Adventures? More than I could count. Challenges? Please. Badass? I'd like to think so. Not because I've done countless battles with one of America's deadliest warriors, but because I never surrendered. I never left him behind. I never gave up on Us.

So, finally, I decided our life would be our life, and that was okay; it really was no one else's business. Not my family. Not my friends. Certainly not my parents. That's how it had to be. We would project a happy life. But that's tough to sustain, so, in order to protect the love of my life, I continued to avoid social settings more than was healthy for me.

I knew I would go crazy if I kept that up forever.

Find Your Oprah

Like I've been saying, it is a key component to mental health that we tell our stories, that we release the toxins before they build to the point of explosion. Knowing this, I purposefully began to work on not isolating myself, even when it would have been so much easier to avoid the eye rolls at family reunions.

I have selected a few trustworthy confidants, people who will not condescend to think they know what is right for me and Tom. My best friend Laura helps me unpack "my stuff" without judgment; without her, I think I might have ended up at the bottom of a cliff somewhere. Not because I slipped, but because I jumped. She will ask hard questions but work through the answers with me. We call each other "my Oprah."

I sometimes would be having such an intense secondary PTSD moment after an interaction with Tom that I'd slink into the back of my closet, crouch on the floor, and pour out my heart and angst in a whisper over the phone.

I could only do this because I knew she wouldn't stop loving Tom. I couldn't bear that. I loved him and I loved her, and I needed us all to be on the same side. Even back during the worst of times, she understood him to be a good man with a terrible condition. No matter what I shared with her, once she knew I was safe, she was understanding and empathetic. I didn't want her to hate him, or even dislike him. Never did she bring that to my door; she just listened and loved.

Everyone needs a friend like Laura. This acceptance from a tribe member is part of the arsenal of tools necessary to heal. I'm lucky, I do have friends who are fun to be around, good for my heart, and loyal through the toughest of times. Another of my best friends, Donna, is more like a sister. I've been close with her with since we were eight. She provides rational thinking and sound advice, there for me in my darkest times.

I am careful not to share the dark bits with those outside my circle, especially those who can be hypercritical or gossipy. You need a tribe, that's all there is to it. If you don't have one, look around. Where are those people who share your values or way of life? Seek them out, at the library, church, music events, writing groups, book groups, military spouse events, therapy groups, they are out there. Pray for your very own Laura. The universe will provide. Trust me.

My tribe saved me. I was often reminded to take care of myself first. If I wasn't going out and having fun or blowing off steam with friends once in a while, then I was no good to Tom. I need to be strong for him and for me.

When I would call Laura after a bad fight, she'd say, "When the bad days outnumber the good ones, then you've got an issue." The good moments between us far, far outweigh any bad.

The Joneses Are Just as Messed Up as You Are

You can't compare a relationship you have with someone who has PTSD to other types of relationships. Maybe you and your partner are that cool couple who can wake up one morning and decide they want to fly to Vegas for the weekend, or maybe throw a spontaneous barbeque for the neighborhood. Tom is not that person. At least not easily, no matter how much he wants to be. He perceives the unknown as chaos and it has to be squashed, immediately. So, I have to put aside my own spontaneous nature and honor his triggers, knowing it's going to be the rare day that we do something without a plan in place first. But I love him and I love Us, so it's worth it to me.

Besides, as the saying goes: comparison is the thief of joy. Images of happy families, happy couples, big houses, exotic vacations, that girl who looks infuriatingly good right after she just woke up, drinking her coffee next to her well-groomed dogs in front of a gorgeous mountain backdrop...Yeah, that can still wear on me. Even though I *know* better. If you invest in comparison and ignore that perfection is a façade, it only deepens the depression. I know, I was there. Some days I still am.

Why can't we be like them? That guy seems so normal. I bet they never fight.

Though I know what really happens behind closed doors. I've heard it all from my clients, but the façade cracked wide open when I was going through my divorce and all the moms who I thought had these great relationships were now confessing quite a different story. Then, instead of thinking everyone was happy and perfect, I started wondering if anyone was happy at all.

Don't worry, I've come around. Happy people are all around us. You just can't compare your version of happy to theirs.

How Grace Got Her Happiness Back

Grace was the perfect image of a high-level Special Operations officer's wife: beautiful, warm to others, involved with the FRG (family readiness group), and volunteered for everything she could at her four children's school. She had a picture-perfect marriage to the outside world, together for over twenty-eight years, always smiling and posing with her family at military ceremonies, and of course, on Facebook.

I met her at a retirement ceremony a few years back, and she and I talked at length about the work Tom and I did with All Secure Foundation and Virago. She talked about how she'd love to get involved and pay it forward with the young wives who don't know what to expect from the rigorous Special Operations tempo.

She shared her story and it wasn't so picture-perfect. She'd done well when the kids were young, although it was difficult managing the house, kids, and their family dog, but she was in a routine and had it down. Luckily, she also had a few girlfriends who had kids the same age, and they spent time together when their husbands were overseas, a mini tribe, helping each other out with school pickups and birthday celebrations, and so she was busy, distracted. But as the kids grew, two now in the service themselves, she found herself with not much to do and not needed by the kids. The empty-nest feeling had settled in before they were even gone, and depression and anxiety crept in around the same time.

As her husband went on more back-to-back deployments or spent his time at home training stateside, she began to question everything. She had spent years as the officer's wife and the home-room parent, but then in her late thirties, her identity seemed to disappear, and she began to spiral down. She noticed the things that used to make her content or joyful didn't anymore, and simple things caused an anxiety response that she didn't understand. She didn't want to meet new people, and most of her girlfriends from when her kids were little had moved to different bases or were no longer in the military community. She felt alone, confused as to what to do next and where she belonged, and, even worse, she didn't know if she still loved her husband.

Well, yes, love, but *in* love? No. Resentment had crept in, for all the missed birthdays, Christmases, and anniversaries, for all the times she had to give up a dream vacation because something came up at work. To make matters worse, when he was home, he wasn't *really* there. She didn't know about PTSD and what was happening with her husband, only that he'd become cold, bitter, and a flat-out asshole most of the time. She had given her life to his career, and while she never regretted it, she wondered where her place was now.

They barely spoke except for when they had to, about the kids, the house, or when he would be gone again. He never talked about the deployments overseas, and she had little knowledge about what went on, therefore feeling left out of the thing that he gave his life to. Disconnected and on the verge of throwing in the towel, she sank further into a deep depression. She was miserable a good three years before she reached out for help. And only then it was because her sister had said, "Enough! It's time for you to put the oxygen mask on yourself. Take care of *you* for a change." Her bubbly personality had turned hard, even cold, and even faraway family had noticed. She didn't know how to care for herself. Frankly, she didn't really value self-care, as her identity was tied to her children and her husband. But mid-life can throw a massive curve ball when you don't pay attention to your own needs.

Brené Brown describes this not as a mid-life crisis but as an unraveling. She says, "The unraveling is a time when you are challenged by the universe to let go of who you think you are supposed to be and to embrace who you are."

When Grace finally went to see someone, she wasn't impressed. Thankfully, she didn't give up and eventually did find a therapist she liked and went every week until it became once every other week and then once a month to only calling for an appointment when she felt she might be slipping, which is normal. When her husband was home from deployment, he would go with her, and, at times, he would see the therapist on his own, to find better ways to manage his PTSD.

They worked together to rebuild the foundation of their relationship and to plan for what they would do in a few short years when he retired. They suddenly had something to get excited and passionate about together. A common goal.

She also found a passion for art and started making things to sell through her own Etsy shop. It was something just for her, and it made her happy to feel she was making things that would make others happy.

She told me she discovered that many of her friends were going through the same thing at the same time, yet no one had noticed. She joked, saying she now calls it the boob factor—a lot of her friends got boob jobs around that time, and now they have all had them removed. Every one of them had hoped bigger boobs would fix the marriage and make them feel better about themselves. That hadn't worked for any of them.

"Just get a push-up bra, don't get the boobs," she told me. "But, in all seriousness, I hope awareness can be built around the deep loneliness that spouses feel, and how, untreated and ignored, it can spiral out of control and lead to more serious situations, like suicide."

Women like Grace are out there. It may be you. You are not alone. Reach out. We got you.

There Is No Such Thing as Perfect

The challenges I've faced since I met Tom have taught me how to be a truly independent woman. While I enjoy being around others, and definitely being with my man, I discovered I didn't need anyone else to make me feel complete or even happy, nor did I have to live up to anyone else's expectations.

But for that epiphany to occur, I had to get a handle on another: I had PTSD. My warrior husband had complex post-traumatic stress disorder. And I had secondary complex post-traumatic stress. Once I recognized the obvious (with the help of my therapist), the researcher in me jumped on the science, getting to know the biology of the condition. The counselor in me got busy with self-analysis, so as to better understand Tom and myself.

Before being married to Tom, I'd always believed an independent woman called the shots; she was confident and self-assured, she never let anyone put her down emotionally or physically, she was bold and self-reliant. According to my domineering mother, an independent woman was in control at all times. She shouldn't rely on anyone, especially a man. In fact, according to my mom, a woman should be the one to wear the pants in the family, as she did in ours. If I was not a confident, self-assured woman, taking shit from no one and asserting dominance in every situation, then I was nothing. And, so, that's how I interacted with others, being the tough broad (though I did try to be polite while being firm), thinking this is what would earn me the respect of others and the approval of my mother.

If I didn't feel this way, I learned to fake it. I wanted desperately to be seen as an "independent" woman, because in my mind that had become synonymous with being the "perfect" woman.

After a few years of maintaining this persona out in public while going through PTSD with Tom, hiding the upheaval and hurt and oppression in my house, my sense of self was really getting ground down.

So, I redefined what "independent" meant to me. My mom was wrong. I couldn't be the perfect woman, because perfection doesn't exist, and it certainly didn't mean that I should be bracingly domineering. I didn't need to act like I was in charge of everything and have a "you damn well better kneel before me" attitude in order to consider myself strong. I am independent because I can choose whatever path I want to go down, regardless of the opinions of others or the past beliefs that no longer serve me. It means having the courage to say "I don't know." That I'm *not* in control every minute. That I can be soft. Or strong. Or sad. Or whatever damn emotion I need to feel at that time. And to love a man means to be vulnerable with him, to be partnered with him. Control is a lie we tell ourselves to feel better about our own insecurities, to create a false sense of safe.

I walk through the supermarket or hang out with friends at a bar now and I hold my head high, laughing or not, chatting or not, being whoever I want to be in that moment. I am who I am. Tom is who he is, and I love that person. I am independent, but I am not perfect, and that is okay.

A Final Note on Social Avoidance

KaLea Lehman, the executive director and founder of the Military Special Operations Family Collaborative, has kindly shared some of her data and thoughts regarding connections. She states, "Broad interdisciplinary research supports that connection is critical to well-being. However, who you connect with matters; there is research suggesting that if your whole network is stressed or drowning, then you will drown faster.

"Being thoughtful with your friendships and confidants is really important for anyone. MSOF has a workshop that addresses the need to seek friends, support, or mentors tied to fitness, family, and personal goals, because when you *intentionally* connect, your network knows you and your intentions. They can then rally to get you there and vice versa, but it's essential to have support for both your family and personal goals. If your network isn't invested in your whole family, then when things get rough, for whatever reason, they won't support your family unity.

"Self-isolation/social avoidance can be an indicator of secondary trauma or compassion fatigue. I think this is relatively common in the Special Operations community, due to the unique military culture and the intensity of the lifestyle. This can put both the service member and family at higher risk when things get rough. This may be a contributing factor in the SOF suicide issue."

The building pressure of pretending everything is perfect at home can take down a military spouse. This is why the All Secure Foundation created Virago, to support women who are in a relationship with either a military serviceman, veteran, or a first responder who is suffering from service-connected PTSD; everyone is welcome. We are a resource for treatments, information, support, or simply a kind word or a shoulder. There is no judgment and zero tolerance for negativity. We are in this together, a tribe of women warriors, bound by trauma but not defined by it.

I stopped aiming for perfection, both in myself and in my home. I have stopped apologizing for my messy parts and beautiful parts and sometimes ridiculous parts—in myself, in in my home, and in my spouse. I've grown. I know now what it means to be a truly independent person and, at the same time, a healthy partner. Avoiding social situations isn't healthy for anyone. Ask yourself why you're doing it.

SEVEN

A Childhood, Interrupted: On Being a Military Child

Military children who have a parent with complex PTSD may develop their own condition, after prolonged and repeated trauma in the house. That sounds so harsh, I know, but this is happening in a large percentage of military homes. If there is a veteran or soldier who is present but doesn't know how to connect, or reconnect, post-deployment or post-service, that disconnect will often lead to anger and even violence in the home. When this is a daily occurrence, secondary complex PTSD can develop. According to the VA, this is a real issue, with the PTSD rates in military children rising, and suicide a major risk.

Of course our warriors don't want to hurt their babies, but between deployment and the battle with PTSD at home, it's happening.

Deployment

If you haven't choked back sobs while watching a clip on the news of an Army sergeant surprising his kid at a football game, or a soldier in camo making it to the gym just in time to be part of his daughter's graduation (my God, I'm tearing up just thinking about it), then you need to check your pulse, make sure your heart is beating.

Deployment beats up any parent. When Tom comes across an old photograph of himself and his son as a toddler, or something has happened with the kids, he'll spiral down, saying, "I'm a shitty dad. I fucked up my kid. I wish I could take it all back. God, I wish I could start over."

Tom had very little time with his son, rarely home due to the demands of the job while during deployed or training stateside, and so never had the opportunity to build a relationship. The only regrets he has confessed to me are, one, hurting me, and two, not having a chance to foster the bond that happens between a father and his child.

I tell him we can't be all things. There is an unreasonable amount of pressure for us to be all things to all people. It's just impossible. That belief sets us up for failure. To be a soldier dedicated to taking out the worst of the worst bad guys, you have to be that soldier full-time. There is little room for anything else, not between training and planning and missions. I remind Tom that he might not have been the best dad, but his son was safe and cared for. Tom *was* the best, most elite soldier, and, in the bigger picture, he was creating a safer world for his children. His choice was tough on him and the family, but it benefited all Americans.

The greater good is often not great *or* good for individuals. His son would agree with that. Children often feel abandoned when a caregiver is not present for long periods, even the older ones who understand what is happening. Another layer is added when the parent left at home has even less time for the child, because that parent is suddenly doing the work of two to maintain the household. And, of course, the threat of death of a parent overseas feels very real and immediate, especially if members of other military families in their life have been killed. Even if the child is too young to know where Mommy or Daddy are, they can pick up the anxiety of the remaining caregiver, and they know it has to do with the missing parent. Kids aren't stupid.

My dad served in the Air Force for a decade, but my mom asked him to hang up his uniform before I was born, unwilling to move to a third town with my brother and sister, who were both toddlers at the time. On the other hand, my older brother moved out when I was ten and eventually went into the Air Force after a stint in college. He set up computer and radar systems for Special Operations. We never knew what exactly what he was doing or where he was. We did know he was in the Gulf during the war, although he never saw battle, and my family didn't seem overly worried. But when he went silent for six months, doing anti-drug cartel work in the Caribbean, it was different. I was fourteen. One night, I woke up in a blind panic and started screaming for my mom.

"He's dead, he's dead, he's dead," I sobbed.

My mom tried to calm me, telling me it was a bad dream, but I wouldn't have it. I knew someone that I loved had died. A man. I don't know how I knew, but I did.

"Is it your brother?!" my mom asked, quiet panic on her face. I didn't know. I made her sleep with me that night, something I hadn't done since I was in kindergarten. At nine in the morning, the phone rang. It was so loud, it startled both my mom and I out of bed. She sprinted down the hall to answer the call. I sat up and listened, waiting for the bad news I knew was on the other end of the line.

Oh my God, what if it is my brother?

I heard her say, "I can't believe he's dead—"

I started to scream, a piercing howl, loud and unrestrained.

My dad came running in to my room. "What the hell?" he shouted, ready to do battle with a murderer. My mom walked in behind him, a hand over her mouth.

My beloved grandfather had passed in his sleep.

"How did you know?" she asked me, shocked and confused.

I didn't have an answer. I was sure there had been a mix-up, that it really was my brother who was gone. It was weeks before I was able to sleep in my own bed alone.

If you're a parent, I'm not saying anything you don't already know. Of course the child's life is in an uproar. Mom or Dad goes away and suddenly little Johnny is wetting the bed again and getting in fights at school. The grades slip, and no one feels like eating. Children don't always have the words to purge the big feelings trapped inside their little chests.

As the parent left behind, it's your job to make sure that everyone who is a staple in that kid's life knows what is happening and that it is okay to talk about it. Let the child process, talk it out whenever he or she feels like it. They don't need to offer solutions or judgments, just listen. Here is where your tribe once again is a boon. The more quality adults who are in your kids' lives, the better. The whole "it takes a village" thing is true, especially when you're suddenly a single parent with a hurting child.

But it's also important that you don't let the destructive behavior slide. You are setting the tone for years to come. If a few conversations with the teacher and a therapist don't curb the inappropriate responses, make sure you are establishing clear expectations, you are role modeling calm and thoughtful behavior (even when you feel like you are going batshit crazy on the inside), and that you seek additional psychological help for the child (and yourself) if necessary.

If you are the parent deploying, set up a regularly scheduled Skype talk and read them their favorite book or look at the moon together, do something that reminds them of the connection that is still there, despite the miles. It is imperative, however, that you work out a plan beforehand with the spouse in regards to a bungled internet conversation—if you have to miss the call because of duty or because the internet sucks, the spouse will need to have an activity or explanation prepared in advance that will distract the child. Otherwise, the missed "date" can add to their fears.

I know there is a lot of literature and research out there on managing children's expectations during deployment. It's so important that you educate yourself if you haven't already. Good places to start are militaryfamily.org or operationwearehere.org. You're not alone, there are people you can reach out to.

Thankfully, kids are resilient. Every parent, even the best of us, has done something wrong. Just ask your kid, they will tell you that is true. My friend's husband, a doting father, was throwing their infant up in the air, because the baby loved it, only to clock the baby's head on a low-hanging ceiling beam. My other friend is a mama bear, and yet she fell asleep and didn't hear the phone ring, so her fifth grader ended up waiting at the school by herself for almost two hours after soccer practice. In the rain.

When a parent has to be away for a long time (and just happens to be shooting at other humans who are shooting at him or her), it can feel like they are doing something wrong with their kids, damaging them somehow. Thank God, the young tend to adjust to a new normal quicker than adults, and love is always in the mix.

But when the new normal means that there is an angry monster in the house, who never seems to leave or to stop barking out orders, that is different. When a soldier comes back from deployment, changed and distant, the child can't just shrug a shoulder and think about something else.

At Home

"Are your kids safe?"

Not an unreasonable question if there is a parent with complex PTSD at home. Let's start with this: if there is any possibility of physical danger, get yourself and the children out of the house. That is imperative. Then, take a breath and figure it out from there. Your warrior doesn't want to hurt the kids any more than you do, not when it's all said and done.

I know the effects firsthand, having grown up with a mother with complex PTSD. The anger, the perfection-driven aggression, the relentless critiques, and the irrational outbursts. It was tough at times. Yet, then, there were the times I would sit on her lap after dinner every night, even jokingly doing that in high school. She taught me how to make the best chocolate cookies, took us on trips after saving half a year to do so, worked harder and longer to send us to private schools, spent weekends at museums, the zoo, and so on. She did her best, and I'm grateful for the lessons I gained from my childhood. It took time, but I came to understand all my experiences, good and bad, and how they made me into the woman I am today. I wouldn't change a thing.

There were very strict rules that Tom and I agreed to before he moved in with me and my kids. He wouldn't be the disciplinarian—that's oftentimes when things went south with his own son. He wouldn't yell or critique, and under no circumstances would he spank or threaten to hit or harm. Five years later, and he has followed these rules to a *T*. My kids have a great relationship with Tom, and we talk openly about what war has done to him and what it means for his mental health. They have never seen an outburst from him. Normal moments of anger, yes; outburst, no. He is able to use the tools he has learned, so, when he gets really angry, he removes himself. He's rarely talked sternly to them. He doesn't really know how to "play" with them, but he tries, and we all love him for that.

This closeness with my kids can be bittersweet for Tom, since the relationship between him and his son is so strained. They barely talk. I can't blame Thomas, who is resentful of the time his father "chose" to spend overseas, and for the anger he brought into the house when he was home, and the constant fighting between Tom and his mother. Thomas struggles with secondary PTSD; at twenty-one, he has just now begun to forgive his father for his trespasses against him and his mother. Tom understands, but we hope that one day his son will find his way to a deeper forgiveness, so there can be a new chapter in their relationship. It's possible. I was much older when I began to process and forgive my mother.

There is an immense peace that comes with forgiveness. Not only for the person you're forgiving but even more so for yourself. Many of our veterans have strained relationships with their children. At All Secure Foundation, we have created a program for reconnecting a combat parent with their child and to help facilitate a healthy relationship between them. Everyone benefits.

Tom is not alone in dwelling on how he was a "shitty" dad. A few times each week, a military parent calls to discuss their "terrible" parenting skills. One call in particular broke my heart. I could feel the man's pain coming through the phone.

"I can't even get on the floor and play Legos, for fuck's sake. I don't know what's wrong with me. He's five and I'm getting mad because he's not putting the set together right. Like that even matters. Why can't I just get on the floor and play with my kid?"

I've heard a variation on this a hundred times. Men can typically find it more challenging to relate to kids or play with them. I suppose it's in part a biological thing, part having their "sensitive" side beat out of them on the battlefield. Yet, I have known many men who are the primary caregivers and do it well, like my own dad or Tom's dad Steve; both men raised their families while their wives went on to college and bigger careers.

I never heard my dad yell once, and he never spanked me. He was the gentle one. So was Steve.

This only frustrated Tom more, remembering his tender-hearted dad. Tom has a huge, loving heart, but he's guarded while his father was effusive. Tom now takes those lessons his dad taught him and holds them close to his heart, often asking himself, "What would Dad do?" when he's needing guidance on how to connect at home. It works, Steve always provides the answers.

Those with PTSD have a hard time not overly controlling the situation, especially when expectations aren't met. I have had calls from mothers frustrated by the delivery of their husband's "lessons" to the children, the harsh tone and expectation of perfection. The ensuing outburst of rage feels so out of place. It's not logical, but that's PTSD, until you consider the fight, flight, or freeze response being subconsciously activated in the soldier. This makes close relationships...complicated.

Tom keeps having breakthroughs, as he understands it better himself.

"Is Greenland a country?" my daughter asked the other day.

"Are you kidding me? What are they teaching you in school?"

She harrumphed and walked off.

It was a non-moment, really. I didn't much take note of it, but, as Tom and I sat around the firepit that night, he said, "I almost got mad at that question, but why would I? She's thirteen, I'm fifty-three. Yet, I keep expecting kids to have the same knowledge and experience that I have."

A lot of his frustration comes from that place: *Shouldn't you know better or do better already?* But, no, a five-year-old doesn't have that information at their fingertips, and sometimes a thirteen- or eighteen-year-old doesn't either. Treating them like little commandos isn't fair to either party, especially the kid.

Depression Symptoms in Children and Teens

You know your child best, but the signs of depression can sometimes be even harder to read in a child, especially a teenager, than it is in an adult.

According to the Mayo Clinic, symptoms in younger children "may include sadness, irritability, clinginess, worry, aches and pains, refusing to go to school, or being underweight." I would also add nightmares, trouble following directions, dreaminess, and getting into trouble at school more than usual.

Teenagers are hard creatures to read. They are going through so many quick physical changes, including the chemical composition in their brains and glands, that the average teen can seem morose and withdrawn in the morning and laughing with their friends by noon. While it is frustrating for a parent, that is completely normal. They hate you one minute and want to cuddle the next (at least, if you're lucky). But extreme emotions or behaviors need to be addressed, or even subtle ones, before they become harmful and persistent. According to the Mayo Clinic, you should watch for "sadness, irritability, feeling negative and worthless, anger, poor performance or poor attendance at school, feeling misunderstood and extremely sensitive, using recreational drugs or alcohol, eating or sleeping too much, self-harm, loss of interest in normal activities, and avoidance of social interaction."

Yeah, I know. Reads like a normal Sunday at your house with your teen and his friends. Just follow your parental gut instinct.

It can never hurt to be vigilant when you know that the child is dealing with loss or trauma.

This topic of secondary PTSD in the combat home needs far more research, and even more programs, in order to support the children effected by their parent's trauma. Not all military children have a parent suffering from complex PTSD in the home, but the ones who do definitely need extra support and care.

When I was fourteen, after years of trauma, I decided that enough was enough, and the only viable way out was death. My suicidal thoughts became daily, and then constant throughout the day. I started to sleep all the time. That was an escape, in my room, alone, and I could be anywhere in the world. My vivid and overactive imagination was my lifeboat, taking me around the world, and also providing me a place where I was strong, confident, liked, and accepted. I came home from high school every day of my freshman year and went to bed. Sometimes I woke up, ate dinner, and then went back to bed. I was severely depressed, suicidal, and trying to make sense of my mother's complex PTSD on my own. One day, I had enough, pressures mounting from a new high school where I once again was being bullied. I pulled my dad's gun out of his lockbox and looked for ammo. It turned out the gun was a collector's item and couldn't shoot for shit, so, thankfully, there was no ammo. Thank God. My parents walked in with me holding the gun, and it landed me in therapy the next day. I went two days a week for a year, and then once a week until I was seventeen. Talking to someone and having them help me sort out what was going on in me and around me saved my life more than once.

You Can't Do It Alone

I mean, you *can* do it alone, but it's not just you who will be suffering, it's also the kids. Whether it's fair or not, the person left behind to care for the children is bearing the brunt of their emotional needs as much as their physical. If you are having a breakdown, so will they.

"The primary caretaker is the one who has the most impact on children," according to KaLea Lehman, executive director and founder of Military Special Operations Family Collaborative. She goes on to say:

"If the mom/caretaker is taking the brunt of the stress—regardless of what it is—protecting the child, and generally thriving, a child likely will thrive, too. Children mimic what they see. They will respond to chaos by distancing, acting out, withdrawing, or other behaviors, depending on their age.

"I believe managing the lifestyle stress—trying to make the frequent transitions normal for everyone—is one reason Special Operations' family culture is so different from conventional military family culture. Most of our families don't draw attention to the fact that they are a military family and especially not a Special Operations family. They sort of normalize a lot of the stress or sometimes trauma by simply ignoring it or downplaying it. For example, they likely refer to a combat deployment as 'away', 'at work', or a 'trip.' You see this behavior less in most other military families because the deployments, moves, and organizational culture almost demand that they recognize the stress and draw attention to it.

"Transitioning out of the service is an incredibly stressful life-change because every aspect of the servicemember's identity, and much of the spouse's, changes seemingly overnight. My guess is, in general, veteran families almost inevitably struggle some. Children are possibly more impacted because there are less opportunities to get a break from stress and change. It's a massive transition that can feel sudden, especially for those in Special Operations, and this stress can really impact kids. Communication, routines, and family support are very important for transitioning families."

If you are new to an area or you find yourself without a tribe, start with the school. They will have a secretary or a counselor who can give you the names and contacts for local services, from after-school care, to child therapists, to family counseling, to financial help or assistance with food for the kids. It means reaching out and asking for help, but your children need you to do that, to put aside ego or embarrassment for their sakes.

It may feel like a thankless job on those long days, when you are trying to finish up a work project while sitting in the car during baseball practice, wondering what you are going to make for dinner when there's a ketchup packet and a box of lasagna noodles in the cupboard…but your kids will know what you've done for them. Maybe not when they're thirteen, but when they get to be adults and understand your sacrifices and hopefully make you dinner once in a while.

One night after a speaking engagement, a young college student came up to me to say hi. He was in the ROTC program and would be headed off to basic that summer. He spoke about his father, who served in Special Operations, and how his goal was to get there as well. But then he switched to talking about his mom, his hero. "My mom is a saint." (Oh, how many times

I've heard that someone's wife, girlfriend, or mom is a "saint.") He talked about how she took care of four boys while his father was rarely home, and, when he was home, he wasn't the best guy to be around. She protected them. He talked about how hard her life was and how much she sacrificed, how much she gave up and never asked for a thing in return. It was obvious he admired her, and, while he was going into service to follow his father's career path, it was clear to me whose shoes he hoped to fill.

Wisdom from Winnie

For kids, PTSD is confusing. Hell, it's confusing for adults; how could it not greatly impact children in the home? It's so hard to explain what's going on and why Dad or Mom isn't behaving like themselves anymore. The warrior may even have come home and then isolated themselves, knowing their behavior isn't appropriate. They end up spending little to no time with the child. Or maybe they go into overprotection mode, or have an expectation of perfectionism, all of which can trigger a violent response.

A.A. Milne, famed for writing Winnie-the-Pooh stories, had a difficult time explaining to his young son, Christopher Robin, about what he experienced with battle fatigue, now known as PTSD. The story goes that one day, Milne was at a picnic and bees came buzzing by, catching him off guard. The buzzing triggered a PTSD episode. His son didn't understand. To explain the effects of war to a young boy, he created a fantastical world. It is theorized that each character explains one of his symptoms. According to a *Military Times* article, "Piglet is paranoia, Eeyore is depression, Tigger is impulsive behaviors, Rabbit is perfectionism-caused aggression, Owl is memory loss, and Kanga & Roo represent over-protection. This leaves Winnie, who Alan wrote in for himself, as Christopher Robin's guide through the Hundred Acre Woods—his father's mind."

Milne wasn't the only author who told stories to explain the complexities of coming home from war. Many believe that J.R.R. Tolkien wrote about realistic war trauma, which was referred to as "shell-shocked" at the time; he began the *Lord of the Rings* series during World War I. His characters were enduring fictional battles in a fictional world, but their responses to the trauma were incredibly real. Another author, C.S. Lewis, was open about the fact that he wrote *The Lion, The Witch, and the Wardrobe* to process his experiences during the war. If it helps your child to understand war and the ensuing trauma, it may be worth picking up a copy of these books and reading them together.

I'm not an expert on caring for PTSD in children, or for children dealing with PTSD. I cannot recommend enough that you follow up with further research when it comes to finding strategies to combat depression or aggression in your child, but, really, more than anything, finding a good counselor is important. If your child uses language that indicates suicidal ideation, seek help immediately. You are your child's greatest advocate, don't wait to get them the help they need.

EIGHT

Magic Pills Are for Fairy Tales: Take Advantage of Multiple Healing Modalities

Tom had turned the corner, committed to getting healthy. I was right there with him.

We didn't have the money for some of the stuff we tried, but we found it. No movies, no vacations, but we knew that getting the right supplements and nutrition into Tom's body was critical or the pain was going to cripple him, physically and mentally, and then we needed to dig deep, get at what was going on in his brain. It was expensive sometimes, investigating different healing methods. At one point, we had eighty-six cents in our bank account after paying for three modalities of healing at once, but we stuck with it because we knew, big picture, this was the only way he was going to get healthy. In the end, our time, money, and hard work paid off.

Did every healing modality work for Tom? No. Did every healing modality work for me? No. I went through three years of talk therapy long before I met Tom. While it helped to have someone to talk to, it wasn't enough to help me fully heal. But until I found cognitive behavioral therapy, I did not get the true help I needed to deal with my childhood and sexual trauma, and then I tried talk therapy again. That's when it worked for me.

A practice called Transcendental Meditation immediately resonated with me, but for Tom, who was still in the thick of his PTSD, it didn't have the effect he wanted it to. Three years later, when he was in the right frame of mind to try again, the technique clicked and worked phenomenally. Just because you try something once doesn't mean it won't work later, or maybe you need to give it ten tries. Spouses and warriors call me, saying, "I tried therapy. I went to a VA appointment. I didn't like it. I'm not doing that again." Really? You went to one fifteen-minute appointment, were disappointed, and now you are going to throw out all types of therapy, all therapists? I had three shitty therapists, but now I have one who is a life- and marriage-saver. Don't give up. Remember when you first learned to shoot? Were you great at it? No, it took a few times for you to figure out how it worked. Even then, it still took a lot of practice to get great.

To get healthy is going to take time and patience and diligence and dedication, and you are worth it. Your life is worth it. Your family is worth it. This community, this nation, this world is better for it.

All Together Now

You've likely heard the term "holistic health." Essentially, it means that when something is wrong with us, we need to assess all aspects of our system, not just the parts. The simplest example is when you are depressed, expending energy crying or letting your mind swirl and swirl, you are also physically wearing yourself down and more apt to get a cold or the flu.

So, when you are thinking about getting yourself healthy, you need to make sure you are addressing all the elements that make up "you"—mind, body, and soul. Each element needs different treatments in order to heal. This is true for all of us, but when a loved one has PTSD tentacles sunk into every goddamn part of him or her, you need to help them use every healing modality available. For instance, eating certain foods and taking certain supplements to make the body strong, sleeping and meditating and maybe even medicating to calm the mind, and therapy and volunteering to help soothe the soul.

I firmly believe practicing multiple healing modalities, which inevitably leads to lifestyle changes, is good for the whole family. If one of you has PTSD, all of you are suffering. These health and wellness suggestions are for everyone, not just the warrior.

Let's Start with the Basics

What did you eat today?

Come on, be honest. If you got up and had a hot pocket for breakfast, diet is going to be a good place to start. If you want to get a handle on your loved one's or your PTSD, you need to get a handle on your family's eating habits. You need all the good energy and vitamins you can get from eating well. A hurt body can't heal if it's not given the proper nutrients, and a hurt body promotes depression and anger.

I'm a certified health coach. I jumped into this particular gig in part because I saw how the Special Operations men and women were beating themselves up physically but not supporting their body's needs necessary to repair the physical damage. Excruciating pain in the knees and the back are common. The joints and tendons can only take so much, and every wound or bullet hole adds up quickly. After a while, the pain is chronic and pain meds aren't cutting it. When it seems like you'll always have this unbearable pain, that can lead to deep depression or suicide.

Tom was in this place physically when I met him. Together, we both turned our health around, committing to a proper diet, guided and purposeful exercise, and supplementing with vitamins and minerals. We struggled with lack of diligence and dedication, and self-sabotage, just like most of you will, but we'd forgive ourselves and keep going. It would have been easy to wake up the day after a night of ice-cream craziness, feeling bloated and depressed, and say "Fuck it. This isn't going to work. I'm meeting the girls for Bloody Marys." And okay, yeah, I might have done that once or twice, but I had Tom and my family to remind me why it was important I not die of a heart attack; I'd jump back into the diet fray.

We have health and wellness programs for veterans available on the All Secure Foundation website. We've helped hundreds of warriors take back their health. But, really, it is a matter of picking a course and sticking to it. If you can't work with us, go online, research eating plans that are aimed at reducing inflammation (that's key) and promote healing. You'll come across a dozen good ones (pegan, paleo, or keto for example). Pick one you can do and go for it. Don't think of it as a diet; I loathe that mindset, which tells our brain that we are giving up something instead of gaining something. The same with exercise or movement. If you're immediately turned off by the word "exercise," reframe it to the term "movement." If you've been out of the game for a while, start out slow doing something you hopefully find remotely enjoyable. A yoga session online or in a studio, or a thirty-minute walk every day or even every other day, is a great place to start. Get a decent pair of tennis shoes and listen to an audiobook or your favorite music. If you can do this for thirty days, it will start to become habit forming. Your body will start to crave that time and you can begin to push yourself. If you're a warrior, you've been here before. Unless the doctor has told you not to be exercising, you got this.

Don't like walks or yoga? Fine. There are a ton of ways to get healthy, like lifting weights, biking, basketball, softball, soccer, surfing...or think outside the box. Pickleball. Fencing. Underwater hockey. Bog snorkeling. Just get up and get moving every day.

Ever eat a bag of chips when you're starving, but you're hungry again ten minutes later? It's because your body is craving nutrition, not calories. Your body is starving for the right stuff. When you fill it with processed foods, you're making your body and mental health worse, not better.

Changing your diet from inflammatory foods to a whole-food diet will change your life; it has for millions of people. In fact, when you have a serious disease and you seek help from somewhere like the Cleveland Clinic, you're going to do just that. People with chronic pain and illness have gotten their lives back by changing their diet and taking vitamins and minerals your body and mind so desperately seek.

Up to 80 percent of our soil is nutrient-deficient, including the soil used to grow the corn in your potato chips. Our bodies need things like sulfur, but the source—cow manure—is no longer used. Since the 1950s, artificial fertilizers are used on crops but don't provide sulfur, so our diets are extremely lacking in a critical mineral. Sulfur is beneficial in many ways, but especially for alleviating joint pain. Once Tom started taking organic sulfur in its pure form, his joint pain was significantly reduced in just four or five days. Vitamins and minerals aren't simply good for you—they are essential for every man, woman, and child.

Most of the guys come to me for nutritional advice at first. Once we get through the food stuff, I happily tell them what supplements to get. You can find a list on allsecurefoundation.org, under the 6 Week Mind and Body Reset, or go to Dr. Hyman's website for a complete list. Yes, it is an investment and, no, you shouldn't go to your drugstore or grocery store to get them. Supplements have to be pharmaceutical high-grade; the other stuff is crap and doesn't work.

After five to ten days of taking high-grade supplements, I would get a call that went like this:

"Holy crap. The pain is damn near gone, and I have the energy of a young door-kicker again!"

Get on a healthy path, not a perfect path, and you will be able to think clearly to get the help you need.

Tom started with nutrition, then his pain lessened, so he got up earlier, worked out more, slept better, had more energy, his brain fog was gone. In a few weeks, so were his depression and anxiety.

I've got a free PDF download on the foundation's website, under the 6 Week Mind and Body Reset. It walks you through supplements, food, exercise, meditation, sleep, and quality of life to help you get jump started.

Finally, find a doctor you trust and go over all of your over-the-counter medications, supplements, and your prescriptions with her or him. *All* your prescriptions. Include the ones you might be buying from online sites or in the gym locker room. Ask for a rundown on the long-term effects of each drug, and make sure you understand how they are interacting. Are you damaging your liver? You need to know. Information is power. Now you can decide which ones to wean yourself off. If there's a narcotic or opiate involved, get out now, but do so with the help of a medical professional.

The flipside is that you also need a good doctor to help you understand what medication you *should* be on. From hypertension, to arthritis, to, that's right, anxiety meds. If you're bipolar but aren't treating it, you are just making yourself sicker. Pull it together. You can do it. Just start now. A month from now, you'll be thanking yourself.

Putting Your Hands to Work

Ever spent a Saturday refinishing a door or putting in a brick walkway? Working with the hands is similar to meditation. If you've got a fix-it project or an art project at hand, you are likely to find that your mind has quieted as your body gets into the slow rhythm of the work.

Finger paint with your kids. Or break out your old oil pencil set and try creating a graphic novel or even some silly cartoon panels. If you like the idea of more long-term projects, take up a painting class at your local community college, or find some old Bob Ross videos on YouTube. If Bob Ross, also a veteran, painting a tree can't calm you down, nothing will. Okay, maybe knitting, which is another great idea and actually very popular among veterans. Don't knock it 'til you try it.

Creative writing is another excellent outlet. Different than journal writing, you are creating worlds and people and conflicts that will eventually be solved. Very satisfying.

In that creative vein, there are local acting troupes in every small town, eager for newcomers to join the ranks. My friend lives in a town with only six hundred people and one cop, a veteran, who just happens to be the football announcer on Friday nights and community theater director on Saturdays. The townspeople love him for it.

Music soothes the savage beast, they say, so maybe it's time you picked up a guitar.

Listening to music is soothing; playing music is a proven method of healing. Singing or playing an instrument has significant power in the process of sorting out emotions and feelings.

A client of mine, Greg, revealed in one of our early phone conversations that he loved music. It was the first time I'd heard a lightness in his voice. He told me he'd been raised playing multiple instruments and that his father was a music producer.

He was newly out of the service and had offers to do contracting work back overseas, but he didn't want that, and neither did his family. Like so many who spent an entire adult lifetime training and working their ass off to do one thing, he didn't know where he belonged in a civilian world now so strange and foreign.

I asked him when he last played guitar. He said it had been years. Special Operations becomes not only the job but the hobby, overtaking activities they once enjoyed. I asked him to dust off his guitar that night and give it a play, even just for five minutes. He called me a week later: playing had set something loose inside him, broke some kind of long-held ball of pain apart.

He felt a love for playing again. How many times do we hear a song and just cry or smile or rage or rejoice? Music is powerful, playing it is especially so. His healing process became more rapid, and although he still had work to do to overcome war trauma, every step in the right direction is a good step.

His wife called me one day and said, "I don't know what you said to him, but whatever it was, it's working. He's coming back. He's doing so much better."

I told her she can thank Gibson or Fender, not me. More importantly, she needed to thank her husband, to acknowledge the strength he exerted to ask for help and the work he was putting in to get better, so he'll be a better man, a better husband, a better father, a better human.

After Greg's experience with music and healing, I bought Tom a guitar for Christmas. He'd played in a band in high school, covering '70s and '80s hits, but it had been years since he'd played. I had never actually heard him play, or even talk about it, until I brought up Greg and his guitar.

Tom started playing that morning and has since played nearly every night, on a guitar that belonged to his father, making him feel a closeness to a man he no longer can call for advice. He plays for him. When he gets upset or angry or just needs to feel, he grabs his guitar and heads out to the deck. Playing gives him peace, it gives his mind something else to concentrate on, it makes his heart happy.

I'm Not Crying, You're Crying

When you're trying to help the person you love but it feels hopeless at times, you search for any and everything to help. We started Tom's many modes of healing first with an addiction and trauma therapist. He was able to help explain anger in a way that Tom had never heard it explained before.

But he was pissed he had to go. It went hand-in-hand with the community service hours he'd been required to complete, thanks to the DUI. "I don't want to see a therapist," he said. "I don't see how they can understand me. They've never been to war."

I asked him one of his favorite comebacks: "Did you go to school to study to be a therapist?"

"Well, no."

My therapist has never been divorced, she isn't a stepparent, and yet she has helped me so profoundly that we folded her into our nonprofit. She has never been to combat and rarely ever worked with veterans, and yet she has helped Tom more than any other therapy or therapist to date.

Therapy has become a commonplace tool for healing, respected in the medical world. The judge required Tom to attend five therapy sessions. He went to ten.

The therapist really listened and then said something Tom has never forgotten. "You're not an addict, you're not an alcoholic. You're a problem drinker. You don't have anger issues, you have PTSD."

Although I had been reading up on anger management, I should have been reading up on post-traumatic stress disorder. I didn't know anything about it, although I had lived with it and with someone who battled it my entire life. Even in someone who had been to war for twenty years, my first thought wasn't PTSD, it was, *Man, this guy has got a serious issue with anger.*

It was the first time somebody let him off the hook. That all of the things that he was experiencing were biological, it was the post-traumatic stress. And when there is a way out of it, there is healing and there is hope. It was the first time he had heard that.

I could hear the relief and excitement in his voice every time he told me about his appointments.

There are many types of therapy out there, not just talk therapy. Don't be afraid to try something you've never heard of, or maybe you've only seen in movies. Recently, we spoke to a hypnotherapist, Philip, who has done extensive work with people from around the world dealing with debilitating trauma, some to the point that they have intense issues living a normal life. One woman he worked with had crippling fears that lead to many phobias. She'd tried every kind of therapy before coming to the hypnotherapist, with no success. She was a severe alcoholic, self-medicating with booze, and no longer was comfortable traveling, both of which greatly impacted their marriage. She no longer was able to accompany her husband on long business trips. Finally, they saw Philip, who in one forty-minute session was able to get to the root of her trauma, which happened to be when she was only six months old. Sometimes, the trauma we battle is subconscious, and it takes something out of the normal to break that trauma free. After decades of debilitating phobias, this woman no longer had a single one. After a few weeks, she no longer drank and was able to travel with zero issues.

In many cases, people entering service already have some trauma from their past. Getting to the root trauma will greatly impact healing from combat PTSD as well.

I'm not saying every therapy will work like this, especially not curing you after one session. As a matter of fact, Tom tried hypnotherapy unsuccessfully, with a practitioner we found out later had no idea what she was doing. We put hypnotherapy on the shelf for another time. Just recently, we met a man from the Royal Marines who had so much success with hypnotherapy that he started a nonprofit to help others get the treatment. And so, like so many things we've tried and found wanting, we will revisit later.

Here are a few other therapies that I know have worked with PTSD sufferers:

- Transcranial magnetic stimulation (TMS)
- Stellate ganglion block (SGB)
- Transcendental Meditation (TM.org)
- Eye movement desensitization and reprocessing (EMDR)
- Hypnosis

- Cognitive behavioral therapy (CBT)
- Emotionally focused therapy (ICEEFT.com)
- Emotional freedom technique (Tapping)
- Prolonged exposure therapy
- Creative art-driven therapies such as music and art therapy
- Equine-assisted therapy
- Anti-inflammatory diet with supplements (allsecurefoundation.org)
- Essential oil therapies
- Sensory deprivation chamber (floating)
- Volunteerism
- Community storytelling / veterans town hall events (sebastianjunger.com)

The Woo-Woo

I was raised Catholic. Although I attended Catholic schools my entire life, it never felt like a good fit for me. Even when I was a little kid, I knew I didn't belong there. I felt a deep connection to the stories of Jesus and God, but the rules that stated how some people belonged there and others didn't was something I just couldn't understand. My mom told me when I was an adult, I could be whatever I wanted, but, in her house, we were all good Catholics. As a matter of fact, she signed me up to be one of the first altar girls in St. Louis, really in the entire country. I hated every minute; it was a stress a little girl already under a lot of stress didn't need. I begged my mom to get me out of it, but this, she thought, would be a great experience for the whole family, to have a family member up on the altar. She was thrilled when the Archdiocese wrote an article about me and the eleven other girls.

As a twelve-year-old, I did as I was told. When I realized it was inevitable, I told myself, *Let's get this over with*—I volunteered to be the first girl to serve. I didn't expect that the day I walked up to the altar, faced a shocked congregation, and delivered the mass, I would have to watch as several people immediately got up and left the church.

I felt it confirmed everything I believed at that time: I wasn't enough. I wasn't worthy. It was a totally humiliating experience. As an adult, I can look back and know that had nothing to do with me or my female adolescent body on God's altar, but some deep-seated fear or resentment in *their* hearts. But tell that to a twelve-year-old. This isn't what made me turn away from religion, but it didn't help.

Yet, regardless, I've always known there is something bigger than myself driving the universe. Spiritual studies are fascinating to me. I love reading everything on this topic, from ancient texts to contemporary practices, from energy work to researching the beautiful American Indian connection between nature and spirituality. I've never had a reason to judge anyone's religious preference; what others believe is, frankly, none of my business, and my beliefs are, frankly, none of theirs.

I believe that everyone has the right to their own belief systems. Belief and faith in the bigger something are powerful, no matter the shape.

When Tom and I started to open our minds to our spirituality, that is when the serious positive changes really started to happen. I am well aware how woo-woo that sounds, having always considered myself somewhat grounded, but I tell you honestly, when I started connecting to the universe, things changed. For Tom, too. The moral injury done to his core essence, that which makes him who he is, was tearing apart his soul and had not yet been addressed.

Back in chapter 5, discussing survivor's guilt and moral injury in depth, I talked about the deeply beneficial effects of helping the less fortunate in your community. Being of service here at home made Tom feel useful once again and soothed some of the guilt that was eating away at his soul. I cannot underscore enough how strong a tool volunteerism is in your arsenal against PTSD.

Some of the positivity of that experience was because he was once again belonging to an organization of people. Spirituality is like that...there is a spiderweb of connectivity between all of us. We just need to find a way to tap into it, to submerse ourselves into the realization that we are not alone, we are tied to one another, lifting each other up, sharing our energy, like it or not, and there is a greater force holding the whole shebang together.

I feel most in tune with this side of my spirituality when I am doing Transcendental Meditation, the meditation technique I mentioned earlier that promotes relaxed awareness, sluffing away all my distracting thoughts and stress as I sit with my eyes closed and generate a silently-made mantra to focus my concentration. TM was created and made popular in the '60s and '70s by India's now-deceased Maharishi Mahesh Yogi and is taught worldwide through a standard course of instruction by trained instructors. The Yogi believed it was necessary for "relaxation, stress reduction, and self-developments," according to the TM Movement, and I happen to agree with them. So does Tom, even though it took him a while to get there.

Thank God he gave it another chance. That daily twenty minutes of focused meditation in the morning now makes a world of difference for him and how he is able to better deal with the triggers that jump out at him throughout the day. Within weeks of the practice, he was removed from high blood pressure medicine completely, that's how powerful that tool is for stress.

To be clear, meditation does not infringe on your religious beliefs, it is practiced globally by members of all religious faiths as a way to reduce stress and to make a deeper connection to your personal belief system. The David Lynch Foundation offers scholarships for veterans and first responders to learn to practice TM; in fact, they gave us a grant to learn the practice. Where there is a will, there is always a way.

If you are struggling with your spirituality, you're not alone. Many service members who were once very religious or spiritual can lose this part of themselves during combat, especially after prolonged exposure to violence. If you would like to step back into spirituality but are uncertain how to do so, there are many books and references (some of which are listed in the appendix) on how to tap back into your connection to God, the Source, Universe, or whatever you call your higher being. Consider going back to church, or maybe even trying it for the first time. And there are many types of spiritual gathering places and events be-yond traditional churches; do some research and find your best fit. There is always going to be a spiritual community who will embrace you into the fold, no matter your trespasses.

Whatever you do, just don't skip this step in healing. Take care of your soul with the same vigor you should be applying to healing your body and mind.

NINE

Love Him (Even When You Don't Want To): Recognizing and Changing Negative Cycles

WHEN TOM IS IRRITATING ME BY BEING A JOKESTER OR A SMAR-tass, maybe even your run-of-the-mill asshole, I will never roll my eyes and say, "Great, here comes Crawler." I'm not going to use Tom's warrior-self as a weapon against him, not even sarcastically. When that side of Tom really does show up, Crawler is mean and unrelenting and no joke.

There were times before I understood where Crawler comes from and that he can be derailed that I didn't want to be in love anymore. Realizing we could break the back of the PTSD if we worked at it together helped me decide to stay, helped me decide to love Tom. Make no doubt about it, it's a choice to show up and love, and I make that choice daily; we both do. It's a choice, not just a feeling.

That realization helped me decide we needed to buckle down and kick this thing into gear. Time to start communicating better, get rid of our bad relationship habits and harmful patterns.

I talked about healing modalities earlier. All of those are helpful in breaking from the negative behaviors that you or your spouse are trapped into. Here are a few more tools.

Tell Your Dark Side to Stop Repeating Itself

As I mentioned earlier, being aware of the dark side of Tom's psyche and what brings him out is key to helping Tom take a breath and corral himself. To call out Crawler when he emerges works for us. To vocally acknowledge that the warrior side of Tom is not needed in a home-life situation is an awareness tool that stops the negative cycle in its tracks.

Tom's got Crawler to deal with, and I've got my Jenny-Jen-Jenna sides busting out in different environments. We are responding to our surroundings by adapting to them, letting different aspects of our personality come forward in certain situations. We all do it, for good or bad.

Well, most of the time. Nothing works 100 percent perfectly, 100 percent of the time.

But defining and naming the different personalities that make us who we are is not new. Tom and I are not the only ones addressing the idea of multiple personalities. Besides soldiers with complex PTSD, there are many military or veteran spouses or children who develop personalities to help with secondary

PTSD, brought on by being traumatized in abusive home situations, or by caring long-term for someone who has been horribly traumatized.

I bring this up again because it is so important. In order to break unhealthy or even violent behavioral patterns and responses, you have to know where those responses are coming from. Sometimes I say something that is super passive-aggressive and Tom will respond, "I think that's Jenny talking." That makes me pause and think about the side of myself we named Jenny. About who I had to be in order to survive during my childhood and about how I can still react from that place within me. I can't tell you enough how powerful this type of awareness is.

If you have PTSD or secondary PTSD, I want you to take a minute and think about what you are like when you are angry or when you are scared. Are your behavior or responses just a heightened version of your everyday self? Or does something change within you? Do you project more of a mean streak or does your body posture become more intimidating? Ask your partner or someone close to you about the times you don't seem like your normal self. Is that enough of a personality subset that you can actually give it a name? Can you separate out that part of yourself and really analyze it, define the benefits and harms of that side of your personality, like what Tom did with Crawler in the therapist's office?

Identifying the pain in our past, then looking at how that pain has manifested in different personality subsets within us, even giving those names…that has completely changed the way Tom and I look at each other. We are complex human beings with complex pasts. No one comes into a relationship pure. This helps us see maybe where the other person is coming from. To me, it helps me change my thoughts and actions when I realize I've allowed a certain side of my personality to take over in an inappropriate way.

At one of our recent Special Operations couples retreats, one of the couples was really struggling. They were having a number of issues with her coming in as the new stepmom. She felt that her husband was keeping her at arm's length from the kids. She also admitted that while she wanted to be a great stepmom, something was holding her back. They kept arguing about the current situation. They kept repeating the same negative patterns of dialogue, getting nowhere.

When our retreat's therapist broke it down in the session, getting the stepmom to really dig into her past and analyze the past issues, behaviors, and responses she was projecting into the current relationship, she had a massive breakthrough. The stories she had been telling herself were completely different than what she'd been saying out loud. She was finally able to see that she was thinking and acting like her inner child, someone whose father walked out and who later suffered abuse by a stepparent. It was like this giant light bulb went off. Her past was playing a role in her current relationship, though she hadn't realized it, and, so, she was trapped in a negative cycle. For both of them, the reason for the behavior was enlightening, leading to more compassion and understanding, and also offering a concrete issue for them to work on together.

When both people decide to put the relationship first, to create an Us, the first important shift is for each of them to stop trying to "win" arguments. As Tom and I had learned, it is the relationship that loses here. When the couple at the retreat had that same ah-ha moment, there was an immediate impact on their closeness and ability to communicate.

Trust in Yourself, in Your Partner

Like Tom and I, the couple had decided to love their "Us" more than their individual selves and were able to break the negative patterns that had been making them so miserable. To get to this point, you have to trust the person you love. You have to commit to having their back, and you have to know that they have your back. No matter what.

I always knew Tom had my back, even when he unintentionally hurt me. I saw this early on in our relationship, even before we were in a relationship and were just friends working together.

When I went on Realistic Military Training exercises, Tom was there from the start. As a co-worker, I had to trust him. He was essentially my handler; he would move through the exercise, and I would follow him. He would put me in places where I could get the best shot. I was used to being in control on shoots, but I had to let go and follow someone else. I was a better follower than I thought possible—I listened to his instructions and never really pushed back. I recognized this wasn't my area, and I respected his knowledge.

I had to trust him to physically protect me. Sometimes we would stand really close to a door charge for a good camera shot, and Tom would have to evaluate the blast radius, overpressure, debris, shrapnel, and make sure that my position was protected. At the same time, he knew I wanted to push the boundaries and get as close as I could, and he respected that. If I didn't trust him to have my best interest at heart, I couldn't get the shot. We also have to trust we are being honest with ourselves and with each other.

Long ago, Tom told me that part of his comfort, part of his security, is being able to read people. It had been life or death for him to be able to read people accurately. As a battlefield interrogator with some of the worst humans on earth, he'd learned a thing or two about liars. He learned about motivation and what people will do for a cause, or if they value their life more than the cause.

Being able to accurately read me was part of his security, though I didn't understand this at first. It's not like we met and he said, *Hi, nice to meet you, by the way I was a battlefield interrogator, so one way I can feel secure in a relationship is being able to accurately read your emotions. If I can't read your emotions, that causes an insecurity, which causes shame and embarrassment, which causes a post-traumatic stress trigger, which will cause irritability, anger, and possibly aggression.*

Eventually, I figured this out, in the process of working with him on our relationship. Enough that I could ask him about it.

His response was, "When you say nothing, you're breaking my meter. Just tell me that you're sad or angry or whatever and then I'll know. If you don't wanna talk about it, then just tell me you don't wanna talk about it. But don't fuck up my meter."

Man, I really respected that. And now I knew he meant when he said, "Don't fuck up my meter."

He meant, tell me the truth so I can know what truth looks like in you.

But then the issue became, if I would tell him I was sad or depressed or angry, he immediately wanted to know why so he could go into fix-it mode. For the first few years, this was our dance—me avoiding and him chasing after, trying to fix me.

We thought about this cycle for a long time, once we saw it for what it was. We were able to define what we were doing in these instances and name our negative cycle. Now we were aware when it was happening and why. With a little bit of work, we pushed through. No longer do I tell him that nothing is wrong when something is. He also doesn't try to fix it, though I have to verbally tell him not to. Our conversations now look something like this:

"Are you pissed at me?"

"No."

"Are you angry about something?"

"Well, yeah, I am. I'm gonna tell you why, but I don't need you to fix it, okay?"

"Okay."

"I'm a little bit mad because something happened at work, and I was dealing with this person and then this happened and it's just really upset me, and I'm trying to work my way through it, but I'll get over it. So, I'm mad, but let's just let it roll…"

And Tom will say, because he can't help himself, being the fixer, "Do you want me to handle it?"

I can reply back, "Hey, remember, I don't need you to fix this. I just wanted to let you know that's what I'm feeling so that your radar knows it's not off when it thinks I'm mad. Because I am a little mad, but it has absolutely nothing to do with you. I'm gonna walk it off, I need this time to myself for now."

And then it's over. I get to stay a little bit grumpy and try to move through it, and he understands that it has nothing to do with him and there's nothing he can do to fix it at the moment. This is a critical step in the daily maintenance of our relationship. Really, any type of relationship can benefit from this analysis, being aware of and naming the nasty cycles getting in the way of open communication and hopefully caring. Find a way to constructively deal with the cycle that you both can agree to, and then practice it over and over again until that is your new muscle memory.

Is this the perfect fix to every argument or negative habit? Hell no. That's not possible. But it helps way more than you can imagine.

Where Do You Live?

When you live in the past, you can't live in the present.

Identity isn't what you do for a living, it is who you are at the core that is the true you. If you ask yourself, "Who am I?" how do you answer? If I say, "I'm a CEO at a nonprofit," I'm defining myself by what I do, not who I am. What if the nonprofit went away, would I still be Jen? Yes, of course. So, then who am I? I'm a wife and mother. But God forbid something happened to my husband and kids, would I still be Jen? Yes. It is not our career, our awards, or any titles we might have, and it's not who we love that makes us who we are. So, then who am I? Who is Jen? Those are questions we have to be constantly asking ourselves. The answer is a combination of all your personalities and connections and experiences. And, honestly, who you are changes all the time.

That's okay. You should be a living, breathing creature, changing and adapting, hopefully for the better.

A few years ago, I got a call from a young Ranger who was having trouble with his transition. He'd been out of the military a little over a year but still couldn't find a place in what was now an unfamiliar civilian world.

I could tell by the language he was using he was insecure in his new community, so different from the military community. He was medically retired due to a persistent injury; he had planned on being a serviceman for his career. The physical handicap had thrown him for a major loop, leaving him in pain and depressed. More so, he had no idea how to create a new identity, so he tried to hang onto the old him, the military guy. He was stuck in the story he was telling himself.

It's something I know well; I do the same damn thing. It's easier, though, to recognize somebody else's worn-out story, which is why I have a freaking awesome therapist, and a spiritual guru, and a friend I lovingly call Oprah. Each of these women make sure I'm keeping it real. When I help someone, it's largely just listening to the story they are telling themselves and then helping them see the pattern of thinking they are stuck in. Again, all I can do is shine the light; they have to decide to do the work.

This Ranger believed he was supposed to live his life as a soldier, and that the only life worth living was as a soldier. Now, living as a civilian with a civilian job was not only dissatisfying but went against the very core of who he felt he was. His identity had been stripped when he was medically retired. Without that specific identity, he felt insignificant, without purpose. He had even lost his tribe, since he'd agreed to move to his wife's hometown, where he knew no one, and his brothers were thousands of miles away. He was in a job that made him feel worthless. I could hear nothing but despair in his voice.

This was a pretty common phone call, sadly. Most new veterans, and some old, talk about feeling insignificant in a civilian role, out of sorts, and displaced in a community that they do not feel a part of, or in sync with. They feel like an outsider at work and even at home. For many, this is because they are stuck in the past, not able to redefine themselves.

This, of course, is not reserved for military service members. I've met middle-aged executives who are repeatedly bringing up high school touchdowns or their college frat years. Unable to let go of who they were in their perceived glory days. Enjoying memories is one thing, finding pride and meaning in who you are now is another.

You have to focus on where you are today and where you want to go tomorrow. It's important to get the story of your past out, who you were, to use your words, talk about where it hurts, and why it hurts, and sort out your feelings. But you can't live there. You can visit, but you can't stay. Build your new home, your new place of being.

A man approached me not long ago at a conference. "I'm a former Green Beret," he said as a way of introduction.

"Thank you for your service. What are you doing currently?"

He looked taken aback. He had left the service nine years ago, but his Green Beret days were the most meaningful he'd had. He was unwilling to find value in who he'd become since then.

"While I appreciate and honor what you did for your country, I want to know about the you now. Start with that. We can get into the past later."

That can feel like a real slap, I know. I don't mean that those days mean nothing now. In fact, far from it, those days should be cherished and honored and held dear to your core. What I mean is you lived those days, you changed as you lived through those days, but you've lived more days since then. So, again, I ask, "Who are you now?"

Going back to the young Ranger, after chatting for a while, I asked him to change his language for one week. The thing I love about talking with military servicemen and women is that they are great with follow-through! He was eager to live a better life. At thirty years old, he had a hell of a long way to go. It would be a damn shame if he lived many more decades, or even just days, holding himself back. It always amazes me that these men and women feel done with their lives at such an incredibly young age, when most people are really just hitting their stride in their thirties and forties.

"I can't call my friends, they're still active and don't get it. I can't relate to my young son, I don't know how to play with him without getting frustrated. I can't take my wife out for a date, we've got too much going on. I can't look for a new job, even though I hate this one, but we need the money..."

Fear was behind every "I can't."

I told him that for one week he couldn't say, "I can't." Whenever he was about to say it, he was to replace it with "I won't."

"I know you are fully capable of moving forward, you're stuck in an insecure cycle. Once you start figuring it out, I know there will be no stopping in you." He was incredibly intelligent, and he'd been highly motivated in the military. If he could apply that to his current life, there would be no limit to what he could accomplish. More importantly, he would have peace knowing that his life's purpose was not fulfilled entirely in the military.

"I can't get on the floor and play with my son," became "I won't get on the floor and play with my son."

"I can't look for a new job," became "I won't look for a new job."

I told him to write down every time he replaced "I can't" with "I won't" in order to find a pattern. What was it that he felt he couldn't accomplish and why? What could he do about removing "can't" from his life?

Most importantly, by tweaking his words, it became obvious he was making choices even in the midst of feeling helpless. If he chose not to get on the floor with his kid, he could choose something else to do with him.

We talked ten days later. I immediately could hear a shift in his voice. The Ranger sounded lighter, happier, and determined. In the span of just a few days, he had taken his wife out for a dinner date, he'd found a way to connect with his son by showing him some basic outdoor skills, and he'd started to look for a new job.

Yet, he still hadn't reached out to his Ranger buddies, and I asked him why he didn't touch base with his old friends. He felt like they didn't want to hear from him, that he wasn't part of the tribe anymore. He was a civilian. Banished from his group of friends who had been more like family.

Never once did a friend of his say anything close to this; he was telling himself a false, negative story. Most of the stories we tell ourselves, the ones that hold us back, are untrue. I asked him, "If one of your brothers was medically retired and they moved across country due to family, would you have totally cut them out? Isn't your brotherhood bond for life?"

He eventually processed his shame and embarrassment over being forced out of an organization he'd been fully committed to for over twelve years, all because of an accident. He'd had to pull his car over on the way home from base on his last day because he was shaking so hard. By him leaving service, he was leaving his brothers behind. Something he vowed upon his life he would never do.

This wasn't something we could solve in two phone calls. This was an issue he was going to have to face head-on, work through, heal from, and come up with a new plan for a life worth living.

We agreed he would reach out to two of his Ranger buddies, a simple text just to say hey. Which he did. Then he realized very quickly that they still had his back, still loved him as a brother, and always would. It didn't immediately fix his issues, but it was a big start. Isolating from your tribe isn't healthy. You need your people in your life, unless they are toxic. This wasn't the case with the Ranger.

You have to do the dirty, hard work to get to the other side. There just is no other way. You can't say you want to be ripped and not go to the gym. You can't say you want inner peace and not heal old wounds. They don't go away on their own, they don't get better by ignoring them; you have to face them, own them. You have to use your big voice and command the old story to go, that it no longer has power over you. Keep saying this until you believe it.

Use your words for good, especially when concerning your new story. If you wouldn't say a nasty thing to a friend, why would you say a nasty thing to yourself? You can survive *and* thrive, if you let yourself. You define your life. You can also define your purpose. Be someone. Be you.

A Story of PTSD

We were hanging out one night with a couple we had just met. Tom and I were telling them about the week before, when some idiots at the house next to us in the Smoky Mountains were shooting off guns, not fifty feet from us, and hooting like morons—and how Tom had not hesitated to mock them.

At the end of the story, the guy we'd been talking to says, "Oh, do you have the PTSD?"

The PTSD, I thought. *Here we go.*

It had been brought up in an earlier conversation that Tom served, but really not much more than "I was in the Army." Tom never tells anyone he was Special Operations, especially Delta Force. He doesn't find it necessary to bring it up, thinks it sounds like bragging, unless, of course, I'm shoving his ass out onto a stage or encouraging him to write a book to help others. He was and always will be the quiet professional.

Tom awkwardly answered, "I'm recovering from it, much better than before, but yeah, I do."

The man said, "Well, that guy shooting guns must have set off your PTSD." Then, his eyes alight with excitement, he continued,

"Did it feel like you were right back in Iraq? What I mean is, did you think you were right back in actual Iraq and taking cover?"

No, my fucking husband doesn't feel like he is actually back in the hundred and fifteen degree Iraq desert, in the middle of a firefight. He's not delusional. When we are at an event and unexpected fireworks go off, Tom jumps and slightly ducks his head. It is a natural biological response. There is absolutely no conscious thought in that reaction. And he hates it every goddamn time he does it. It embarrasses him. He hides it quickly or passes it off with a joke. He hates that his mind and his body still respond like he is at war, but this is not some sort of conscious show of trauma. There are many people who fabricate war stories in order to get attention; I've met many, many of them. And there are many, many who fabricate PTSD, and act out what they think it looks like. It always stands out as false or funny to us and to most around them.

My husband doesn't want to have PTSD. And we work hard so that one day he will no longer have it. He is light-years ahead of where he was seven years ago. However, fighting the biological response is tough, like when I gripped the steering wheel subconsciously for a few months every time I sat at the stoplight where I'd been in an accident. He will jump or duck when he hears something that sounds like gunfire. That is an unconscious biological reaction. No, he doesn't feel like he's back in Iraq—he heard a noise that his brain told him could be dangerous, so he braced himself. Period.

It's not to say that some people don't have powerful flashbacks, some that can be utterly debilitating and frightening for all parties involved. But those are less common than the biological responses we most typically see as the brain tries to fill in the story.

The Stories Tom and I Tell Ourselves

As Tom and I sat on the porch of the cabin up in the hills of the Smoky Mountains, we took in the sunset with a drink and a long conversation.

We were talking about how the stories we tell ourselves make an imprint at a subconscious level. How those stories sometimes get in the way of what we want most. For Tom, what he craves most is peace and happiness.

We have a choice regarding how to handle those stories we keep dredging up, the ones that are hurtful and keep us in a negative cycle. We need to tell those stories again, but re-explore them. Then, when we are at peace with them, we can put them up on a shelf. Leave them be for a while. No need to sit with a hurtful story day in and day out. What good does it do you? Does that one story define all of who you are and can be? No.

Our stories remind us of our experiences, and our experiences help shape who we are. The good, bad, ugly, all of it. But one story doesn't make a person. And when the worst stories repeat in a way that keeps us from living in the now or make us react in a way that keeps us from loving our lives, we have to do the work to put those stories up on the shelf.

For a long time, the story I told myself most often was that I was a victim. In order to no longer be a victim, I had to overcompensate and be a tough girl.

Without my experiences as a child, I wouldn't have developed a victim mindset, nor would I have then developed the extreme sense of will to overcome the impression that I was a victim (which is how I thought others saw me, since that was how

I saw myself for so long). These experiences and responses made me who I am now. Yet, I am not that passive child anymore, nor am I domineering, like I tried to be in my twenties. I am more.

I backpacked in Europe at nineteen with Donna, jumping on trains in France and Spain, trying to prove to everyone I was independent, that I could take care of myself. I lived in London by myself for a time, when I was twenty-one and I'd just finished school in Canterbury. I was no victim, not anymore; I was strong and self-reliant. No one had to take care of me. When I was afraid, I would remind myself I could do the hard things. And I did. I continue to. But the difference between me now and me in my early twenties is that I'm at peace with the experiences that led me to think I was a victim. I've forgiven my trespasses and those who trespassed all over me.

The day I was able to put the story of the abuse on the shelf was the day I was truly free, free to forgive and to move forward. Recently, Tom asked if I thought I still had PTSD from the childhood experiences.

"No, I don't have it anymore," I said. 'The symptoms are gone and all that's left is the story of what happened, but it's been drained of its power to hurt me. Am I changed because of what happened when I was a kid? Yes, but I'm better for it. Stronger. For that, I have gratitude. With gratitude, I have peace."

It took years, but I tell myself now that I was a victim to someone else's choices, and I was hurt, but I didn't become a permanent victim. It in no way defined who I was, or who I am, only that something happened to me. I now tell myself I am a champion of this obstacle course we're all on.

Tom and I talked about it for a while, the stories that took place, the stories we tell ourselves, the stories others have about us, which, of course, is an utter waste of time to worry about.

Then I asked him, "Can you put the Somalia story up on the shelf?"

He sat quietly. In his head, there was sand and blood. "No. No, I can't."

"Then you need to finish writing the story, it's not complete. You have to finish it."

"Yes, I do," he said. A wave of peace fell over his face. "Yes, I do. I don't know what that looks like exactly, but yes, I do."

"Do you worry that if you are able to put away that story, you'll be dishonoring the memory of your fallen brothers? Is that part of it?"

Again he sat and thought. He didn't know quite how to put it in words, but he didn't have to. I could see it in his face, the heaviness of that story, so deeply embedded into his heart and mind, he didn't know how to make sense of it. And the only person that can is him.

"No," he said, finally. "I have done my work, and I don't ask 'why not me' anymore. I could've just as easily been killed. Hell, there were bullet holes in my clothes. I *should* have died; I don't know how I survived. But I didn't kill Gary or Randy, Tim, Matt, Dan, or Earl. The Somalian rebels did. And they tried to kill me. I'm not at peace with my brothers' loss, only that it could have been any of us that day."

PTSD has often been explained as the brain looking for the end of the story. The brain writes the beginning, the middle, and continues to search for the end. That search for closure creates the

PTSD response. Real life rarely has a satisfactory closing to any issue or experience, we don't live in a neatly laid-out storybook. And when the amount of horror that Tom and other warriors suffer through seems to have happened for no understandable reason, with no good ending, then their brains go on overdrive trying to solve the problem.

I think everyone should write their stories down, even if it goes no further than their laptop or notebook. There's something powerful about putting words on paper. But nothing is more powerful than sharing your story with someone else. Tell it until you can see it without crying anymore. Just as Tom had to do.

For Tom and the battle in Mogadishu, Somalia, his brain tells the story, but it never ends. He will end that story one day, though, when it's time. He's getting closer, now that he has finished his book, *All Secure*, and he's told his story countless times in front of audiences for our foundation.

He couldn't talk about Somalia without breaking down, but now he has shared the story so much, he has made peace with a large part of that complex narrative. This is a version of exposure therapy, which veterans or people with trauma have found useful. You tell the story of your trauma over and over and over and over again, until it no longer bothers you to tell it, usually in the privacy of a therapist's office. Tom has stood in front of a thousand people and bared his soul. That takes guts. That's bravery. Most of all, that is vulnerability. We have to be vulnerable in order to heal, grow, love, and live. Vulnerability is courage.

TEN

Pandemics and Race Riots: First Responders, Virus Victims, and Veterans Facing Social Stressors

I WORK WITH SERIOUS, VERY COMPLEX PTSD ON AN ALMOST daily basis, so when it became clear that a global pandemic was going to put a stranglehold on our healthcare workers, I jumped into help mode. I've been reaching out to whoever I think it will help, to share my knowledge about coping with trauma.

But about one month in, when I interviewed the virus PTSD counselor at a major American hospital, I was still rocked to my core. The distress rolled off this incredibly brave and strong woman in waves. Speaking in anonymity, this is what she had to say:

"I deal with almost every single virus patient that comes into our hospital, as part of my job. I'm overwhelmed these days with the things I'm exposed to. We all live in what we call 'swamp masks' for eight, ten, twelve hours per day. And that's just our work hours. We are caregivers and can't even hug our patients or their families, we can't soothe them with needed human touch. Or our own families when we are home—we can't touch them. That is really tearing us apart the worst.

"Decent healthcare people truly love not just *what* we do but *who* we do it for. And this constrains us in ways we've never experienced. On top of struggling to save them. The sheer creativity we've been forced to use is staggering, even though we are known for that at my hospital. Honestly, if I had to talk about this in detail for long, I wouldn't be able to go to work.

"I see perfectly healthy civilians acting like spoiled children over being asked to wear a mask in a store—and we are wearing them even when we eat our lunch at work. These selfish people are the reason we are still dealing with this daily. They come out and clap for us and go on FB and thank us, and it's hypocritical. The best cheering would be to not cause more sickness.

"Someday, I just want to be able to have the same freedom all of you have. To be able to go inside one of those open restaurants. But I still can't. I still can't get a haircut. I still can't take my pets to the vet. Because I'm directly involved with virus people every day. Right now, we medical people live every moment with PTSD, if for no other reason than that many citizens don't believe that this is more than a flu. I foresee many medical folks retiring or changing careers or committing suicide after this has passed. And most Americans will still not quite get why their impact or lack of compassion for others around them is so profound to us and those they affect."

Imagine. Since this interview, she's endured months of nonstop pressure. COVID-19 is causing trauma she didn't see coming. Our healthcare providers are going to be dealing with the emotional and mental toll for years to come. A variation of this woman's story is told daily around the world, often in posts or videos from nurses or doctors pushed to the point of exhausted tears. Most major hospitals are understaffed and overfull at the best of times. For many, post-traumatic stress has already set in, but there are few mental health workers available to support them—or, as you just read, the mental health worker is just as traumatized.

My hope is that the healthcare workers and first responders working with the sick are reaching out to their tribe for support, as well as therapists or counselors. That they are making sure to eat foods high in nutrients and take good vitamins and supplements, and to get some kind of exercise every day, hopefully outside, even just for five minutes. Vitamin D is so important. And sleep is imperative. I know how hard it is to fall asleep when your brain is whirling around, but melatonin or soothing sounds can help, or even a hot bath, a cup of chamomile tea, and reading a funny novel. Remember, your oxygen mask needs to go on first. Take care of yourself if you want to continue taking care of others.

Please, just be safe out there. The sooner we can get the pandemic under control, the fewer PTSD cases and suicides.

Catastrophe, Ain't It Grand

"If it isn't one thing, it's another." That saying doesn't cut it anymore. "If it isn't one thing, it's ten" is so much more accurate. Every single month in 2020 has introduced something new, bringing constant upheaval. These ongoing twists and turns do two things: bring people together and tear them apart.

In Sebastian Junger's *NY Times* bestselling book *Tribe* (2016), he describes how one observer during the London Blitz later studied communities responding to "calamity" and determined that "social bonds were reinforced during disasters, and that people overwhelmingly devoted their energies toward the good of the community rather than just themselves." They worked together in order to survive. Even though the U.S. feels like it is being torn apart right now, we are seeing this kind of bonding within neighborhoods. People are reaching out to their neighbors to make sure they are safe; they are working to protect their local tribe. We may not be unified as a city, or a borough, be we do still have the people around us.

During the initial breakout of COVID, people *were* unified on a bigger level, singing from balconies and cheering health workers after every shift. There was this underlying feeling that *this sucks, but we are all in this thing together.*

Then, within a few weeks, we started getting more stressed, more isolated, more challenged with things going on at work and at home. A pressure cooker of intense emotions and insecurities, including, *If I get this, I might die.* Businesses closed. People were still out of work with no idea when they would go back, if ever. People were dying alone in hospital beds without the love of their families. It was, and still is, horrific. And it is more than our brains can take over an extended period of time.

Early on, most of the people I talked to were keeping it together. In fact, a few people I knew saw it as an opportunity to exit the rat race for a while. *Hey, I'll get my house projects done* and *I'll actually get to spend more time at home with my kids.* Despite how overwhelming it feels at times, there has been good to come out of the government and public shutdowns. People are having massive awakenings in their lives, in big ways.

For example, many have realized that the toxic people in their lives, who they have not interacted with for months, don't actually need to be involved in their personal lives. And the job they hated may not be so hard to leave behind now. The daily lunches out and expensive coffees aren't as necessary as they thought. Baking bread isn't as hard as they thought it was. Long periods of quiet were irritating or maybe even scary at first, but now they've learned to settle into a slower tempo and peaceful moments, and they are hoping they can maintain some of this when the pandemic is over and we "get" to return to normal.

As many calls as we received from stressed veterans, especially in the beginning, there were also lulls that we hadn't seen at our foundation since it was founded over three years ago.

Unfortunately, we've now dealt with this for so long that the benefits are starting to lose their charm. The good that has come from simplifying life will hopefully become habitual, but in the present state of continuing to deal daily with the harmful affects of COVID, the stress has reached a tipping point.

After maybe five or six weeks of relative quiet, we suddenly had a massive influx of calls, emails, and online requests asking for help or resources. Veterans and soldiers at home with their families for long stretches found themselves under duress, with no escape outlets. Add to that the loss of jobs and unknowable futures, our warriors were in Hell. Healthcare workers and those who had suffered traumatic loss due to COVID were calling, seeking answers. For those whose PTSD had already been out of control, the prolonged stress of COVID was the straw that broke their back. We've learned of several Special Operations active duty and veterans who committed suicide since the outbreak. No one can ever know for certain, but we are assuming that the pandemic was influential in this decision.

And then the race riots broke out. Our phones started ringing even more. Civil unrest for so many who have fought overseas is a massive PTSD trigger. It feels like the chaos overseas, but there is no outlet for the anger, for the situation that is completely out of control, and a soldier at home has no power in this type of situation to regain that control.

We are now seeing even more calls for help, more violence in the home. These cries for help aren't just from military folk.

There are the police officers and the first responders out in the streets, accosted daily, just trying to do their jobs, protecting everyone, even those who don't deserve it. Or the peaceful protesters desperate for necessary social change but are being attacked by violent agitators who are turning the protests into riots, usurping the message, or sometimes by the police, who are struggling to tell the difference between peaceful protestors and the anarchists and are overwhelmed and afraid for their lives. There may be violent cops and violent protestors, but the majority of the people out there are just trying to do what they think is right, and they are paying for it.

If you find that you are dealing with symptoms of PTSD, you need to remove yourself from the chaos, ASAP. Get away for the weekend. Reach out to your friends, have a Zoom party, or a socially distanced barbeque. Do not sit and dwell. Spend some time creating a list of the positive things in your life, or think about what you realistically can change to make your life easier, from bringing a sack lunch to work instead of trying to find a peaceful diner, to moving to the suburbs. Above all else, reach out to a counselor (do a search for a counselor who uses Zoom or Skype sessions, there are thousands, and you can see someone quickly and for less than face-to-face sessions). PTSD is not going to resolve on its own. While you may be putting yourself out there for the greater good, the loss of your mental health in no way benefits the community. No matter what you say, it just doesn't.

One piece of advice we like to give is, if at all possible, take some time away up in the mountains or in a little beach town, far away from the violence and chaos in the streets. With your family is great, if you think you can do that safely. Is there a place you can go that is quiet? Ask your friends. There's usually someone who's got a family cabin somewhere. Just be realistic about the risk of too much isolation. If a person with PTSD is alone and there is a chance of suicide, then this isn't a good idea.

History has taught that we will settle back down, for good or bad. At the very least, we will develop a new sense of normal. Humans will find balance in their lives again. We just have to be conscious of what we are going through and how we are responding, and then responsible enough to do what it takes to find stability.

Your PTSD Affects Everyone

COVID-19 has reminded me in a very personal way that my PTSD affects not just me, but everyone around me. If I'm going to continue to fight to keep the symptoms at bay, my family is the biggest reason why.

I was struggling. Being inside and isolated for over sixty days due to the pandemic was starting to get to me, affecting my day-to-day life. My old depression had resurfaced. Maybe because the stagnation of the Groundhog Day we were all living became too predictable for my personality type. I love change, I love breaking from routines, and I love seeing people, so the COVID isolation has been a gut punch. But this self-pity made me mad at myself, considering I have a beautiful house with beautiful gardens and places to hang out, we have hiking trails at the end of our street that go on for miles, and, most importantly, I have my best friend to talk to and my husband and my children with me. I was still working full-time, like I always had from home, so that wasn't any different. In fact, the All Secure Foundation was busier than ever. I was pissed at myself for feeling sorry for myself.

But, logically, I knew what was happening. So many people were feeling the effects of the isolation and upheaval to their daily lives, mentally and emotionally, even those who had no previous issues. Or those who had past traumas they'd thought they were on the other side of but were now facing a resurfacing of symptoms, sometimes in small ways but sometimes in major ways.

The outside world was crazy, but nothing big had happened for me regarding the pandemic, no massive drama or huge event. Tom and I were getting along well, despite having the normal little argument sometimes. Frankly, I have come to accept that living with Tom can be hard, but being *without* him is not the kind of hard I want to go through.

So, why was I feeling so restless and out of sorts? I was becoming more and more tired, listless, without energy; even the daily walks that I normally looked forward to had become a depressing chore. I had to force myself to go, or Tom would have to goad me into it—which I'm glad he did, he knew I always felt better afterward. The woods are a place I can restore myself emotionally and spiritually, syncing myself to the positive energy of the earth on our trails, climbing over rocks, walking through streams, hiking up hills, picking wildflowers. Believe me, I know how absolutely blessed I am to live this close to nature.

Things I normally enjoy weren't interesting me.

All the symptoms that I go over with other people daily were showing up in me. Isolating, depression, lack of interest in things previously interested in, tiredness, irritability, and no motivation to do anything but eat a lot of cookies in bed, watching a lot of TV. Too much. My sleep was crap. Tossing and turning every night, I was waking up completely exhausted, irritable, after having vivid, strange dreams. I woke up every morning with anxiety. I had this feeling like there was so much to do, but I couldn't figure my way through it. I felt out of control, I guess.

Yet lacking the motivation to do anything about it, which in turn was making me feel depressed.

"You gotta snap the fuck out of it," Tom told me.

I looked at him. He had a shit-eating grin on his face. I knew he was razzing me, but he meant it, too.

More gently, he said, "What's wrong with you? What's going on?"

"Nothing."

"Don't fuck up my radar," he told me.

I laughed a little. Tom hated when I fucked up his radar, as you know.

We've talked a lot during COVID about how we are feeling, checking in with each other, checking in with our children; everybody seems to be doing generally pretty well. Like for so many, at first it was a nice change of pace, no travel, a lot of time with the kids, and teenagers that actually wanted to hang around us somewhat. Tom and I work the foundation from home, so it wasn't so drastic for us. However, I'm an extrovert, an ENFP, the most introverted of the extroverts, so part of me was bothered by lack of socialization. I tried to ignore that side of myself and take the time to decompress, to focus on my inner self.

Yet, despite this desire, I struggled to think straight. My brain couldn't settle down. I started growing ashamed over all the projects I thought I would do, including writing this book, but left it sitting on my desk day after day. My lack of follow-through was frustrating and confusing, which just deepened my depression.

What I hadn't taken into consideration was that I was working more hours, with the pandemic ramping up and the increasing amount of people needing help. Not just veterans, but first responders and people in the medical field.

We felt like we couldn't say no to anyone, so we were working seven days a week, sometimes early in the morning until late at night. Taking call after call, listening to story after story. Being invested in each and every person means you are emotionally exhausted by the end of the day. I felt immense satisfaction at the lives that I'd touched and grateful for the positive impact they had on my life as well. Yet, I had failed to put on my own oxygen mask.

While we were getting others help, I forgot to help myself. It's not something I tend to pay a whole lot of attention to, anyway, and it's caused me to end up in a pretty bad emotional state more than once. When you're in the thick of it, though, it's hard to pull out and see the big picture. I didn't even consider that I was emotionally burnt out. I just kept taking the next call and the next meeting and the next Zoom and the next video therapy session. Sometimes I spoke with a veteran or a spouse for two to three hours, and it would be very emotional. It's not like you can cut it short and say, "Hey, I understand that you're in a lot of pain, but I gotta get dinner on."

We had a lot of late dinners, a lot of frozen burritos.

I was failing to follow my own advice. Isn't it funny how that happens? You can tell people all day long how to live their best life, and then you ignore the very advice that you know works, and you wonder why your life isn't going the way it should be going. Knowing isn't enough, you have to do and do, over and over again, and self-care is something I need more practice at. Self-care is not muscle memory for most of us.

I didn't really see this until I had a phone call with my long-time friend and spiritual energy practitioner, Sara. We talked about what was weighing on me. I admitted that the years of working on my own PTSD have been so profound and productive that, as I'd told Tom, I'm mostly on the other side of it. At least, I had been. In these stressful times, symptoms were reemerging.

I told Sara that sometimes I would feel a deep sadness, a sense of hopelessness that would wash over me but didn't tend to linger. Now, however, that sad hopelessness was happening all the time. I couldn't quite put my finger on it. There was also an overwhelming feeling that I was failing, that I wasn't good enough to be doing the work that I'm doing, that I'm a poser. A fake. This type of insecurity was nothing new, I'd felt this way sporadically over the course of my life, but now it was showing up in the mirror daily.

I so desperately, with every ounce of my being, want to help heal warriors, and their families, or anyone with PTSD, but, even after all my years of research and practical experience and trial and error and successes, I knew the war within wasn't over for Tom. And I didn't know how to end it. I felt like I should have the answers by now. By trying to write a book about what I knew worked, I suddenly felt like a failure. How could I pass myself off as an expert? How could my knowledge and experience be enough? I hadn't wholly cured anyone yet, not even Tom. It was a massive ego struggle, a battle with old insecurities, and they were winning.

I told Sara, "I can't save them all. Maybe not any of them. I really want to, but I'm terrified I can't save them. I don't know what to do, I feel so lost sometimes."

As I paced around my backyard, she told me something that made me stop in my tracks. "You're not supposed to save anyone's life. You don't have that type of power. The only life you can save is your own. They have to save their own lives."

I was listening closely now.

"Think of it this way. It's like you're this tall, beautiful lighthouse filled with a powerful shining light, and there are men and women out in rafts in the pitch-black ocean, and you are the light bringing them to shore. But they still have to row to get there. You can shine the light, you can be the awareness, but they have to do the work. It is not your job or duty to save anyone, because the answer is that you simply can't."

The words were a gift. The weight that had been sitting on my shoulders was immediately lifted. I knew in my gut she was right. The weight of others' souls was not mine to bear. I let go.

After speaking with Sara, my depression lifted, my motivation was through the roof, I was sleeping better with no disruptive nightmares, and I didn't have terrible, unshakable anxiety. Instead, I woke up alert and rested, ready to work. I felt recharged. I knew how I could be of service to our warrior community. No longer did I feel the weight of having to save a life. I knew that if I could just shine a light, help them see their way forward, and provide awareness, some hope, and some ways to start them out on their own journey, I was doing my job. If I could offer this knowledge and experience and prompting, then I had done my part. I came to peace with that. We are each meant to have our own experiences. To have our own journey. To learn by doing. Me trying to put in the work for them was robbing them of the experience of true personal growth. I see that now.

I tell you this for a couple of reasons. One, all of us need to hear: we cannot force someone to save themselves. We cannot force them not to drink or not to be violent or to not hurt themselves. We can only shine the light on the path forward for them and offer a hand along the way, give them someone to hold onto when the ground gets shaky. If you have a loved one suffering with PTSD, you must take this to heart. Do what you can and then let go. You are not a savior. You are a partner, as long as that person will allow it.

Two, if you have PTSD, read this again. The answer is within you. Your loved ones or a therapist can help, but you have to choose to step into the light. It is not someone else's responsibility to make you whole. There will always be someone to hold that light for you, if you look around, make the calls, reach out, but the choice to get better is ultimately yours. Accept the help that is given. You can do this. I know. I've seen it. I have faith in you, my friend.

After the call, Tom immediately noticed my mood was much better.

"How you feeling now? You okay?"

I had just finished brushing my teeth and reached over to grab his hand. I looked into his eyes, intently. After a deep breath, I said, "I'm not supposed to save your life. I know that now."

He was stunned but quiet.

"*You* are supposed to save your life, Tom. I am supposed to be your lighthouse. I know you know that, but I didn't get it until just now."

I didn't have to explain any further. He squeezed my shoulder, and we both smiled. A tension between his eyes disappeared.

My reemergent PTSD symptoms over the past months had been weighing on him. My response to his PTSD had also been weighing on him. His shoulders dropped in relief, knowing my shoulders were no longer bowed under an invisible weight. I could see it as his face relaxed, how my pain had been worrying him, digging at him. We hugged each other for a long time.

Just because you want someone to heal doesn't mean that they will. Just because you love someone so much it feels like you can break, it doesn't mean that love is enough to save someone. Because it isn't—not unless the other person chooses to let themselves step into the light of your love. As much as I wanted to save Tom, with everything in my being, as much as I love him, as much as I want him to be happy and well all the time, he has to want it just as much or more. He has to put in the work. By me trying to control his journey, trying to push him or pull him down certain paths, that wasn't getting us any closer to healthy. I wish I had learned this when I was much younger, that when you try to control the outcome or control the path of healing for someone else, you're not allowing them the journey or the lessons they need to gain.

"I'm so relieved," he said. "I didn't really get it until now. The pressure of you wanting me to heal was an additional stress, your stress on top of mine." Feeling like he couldn't heal quick enough for me sent him into a shame spiral, which would send him into an anger fit.

So, I've tried to remove this control factor, loving him instead of trying to control his journey. I'll continue, though, to always be his lighthouse.

Our relationship has grown even closer. He knows I have my own journey and I know he has his own journey. We will take turns holding each other's rucksacks when we need to. That I can do. But I know sooner or later, I'll have to give it back to him. And he will have to give mine back to me. I'll be there, he'll be there, because both of us choose it.

And I'm not just okay with that, I'm great with that.

APPENDIX

Further Reading

For an updated list of organizations, government agencies, academic research, and contact information, please visit our website: allsecurefoundation.org

PTSD

The Body Keeps the Score – Bessel van der Kolk, MD
War and the Soul – Edward Tick, PHD
On Killing – Dave Grossman
Tribe – Sebastian Junger
All Secure – Tom Satterly

Personal Growth

The Gifts of Imperfection – Brené Brown
Braving the Wilderness – Brené Brown

Judgement Detox – Gabrielle Bernstein
The Universe Has Your Back – Gabrielle Bernstein
The Four Agreements – Don Miguel Ruiz
The Seat of the Soul – Gary Zukav
The 5 Second Rule – Mel Robbins
Food: What the Heck Should I Eat? – Dr. Mark Hyman
It Didn't Start with You – Mark Wolynn

Marriage

The Seven Principles for Making a Marriage Work –
Dr. John Gottman
The Science of Trust – Dr. John Gottman
Created for Connection – Dr. Sue Johnson
Hold Me Tight – Dr. Sue Johnson

ACKNOWLEDGMENTS

To the men and women who have so bravely answered the call to serve and protect, to fight against terror and injustice around the world, thank you.

To military families, thank you for your service, sacrifices, and being the duct tape holding it all together. Your contribution to this nation is vital, yet largely unrecognized. I see you. And I thank you.

To my forever tribe, my kids, Luke and Claudia, thank you for just being amazingly you: wise, kind, supportive, funny, and generous with your love and massive hearts. You inspire me daily and make me want to be the best person I can be. Never stop reaching for your dreams, I believe in you and I love you to the moon and back.

To my parents, George and Linda, thank you for the lessons, the ones you taught me and the ones you allowed me to learn on my own. I'm forever grateful for your love, support, and for always believing that I could make a difference in the world, just like you always strived to do. Thanks for showing me that one person can, in fact, make a difference.

To my people, my band of weirdos who have loved and supported me through thick and thin. No doubt we were all sisters in a past life, and I'm glad you're on the journey with me in this one. Thank you especially to Laura Kelly, Donna Stamp, Shelly Aspenson, Sara Ford, and Jamie Hope. And to Stacey Stone, the magical unicorn of healing, thank you.

To Holly Lorincz, my incredible co-writer and soul sister. This book wouldn't have been possible without your incredible talents for taking my pages, voice recordings, and long-ass text messages and turning them into something that will help others heal. Your passion and heart for this book has filled my heart with much gratitude, more than you know. Thank you.

Thank you to my editor, Debra Englander, for believing in this book, and the team at Post Hill Press, especially Heather King. And to my literary agent, Chip MacGregor, thanks for taking on another Satterly manuscript, you have been instrumental and a friend in this process, I can't thank you enough.

And last but not least, thank you to my incredible husband, Tom. Your bravery in this new civilian world, putting all of yourself out there to help others, outshines even the incredible bravery you demonstrated on the battlefield. Your love is so wonderful and big that it helped fill in the cracks in my seams. You are my heart and soul, this life and next.

ABOUT THE AUTHORS

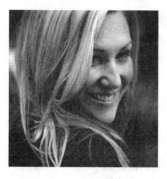 JEN SATTERLY owned an advertising and film/photography studio in St. Louis, creating award-winning work for over ten years. Jen has a passion for service and worked with several nonprofits, including Pujols Family Foundation, where she spent time in the Dominican Republic on a medical relief mission as the documentarian. After years in advertising in the commercial sector, Jen helped to form an elite Special Operations military contracting company as Director of Film and Photography. Jen embedded with and filmed Navy Seals, Green Berets, and Army Rangers on large scale Realistic Military Exercises for over three years.

While working with Special Operations Command, Jen saw a serious need for PTS recovery and became certified as a health coach to better understand the role nutrition, mental health, and emotional health played in healing from the invisible wounds of war. Jen immediately began to donate her time and efforts to hundreds of Special Operations veterans and their spouses to regain their health and combat the effects of PTS. Jen, along with her husband Tom, cofounded All Secure Foundation to serve the Special Operations warriors and their families. She serves as co-CEO.

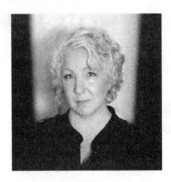

HOLLY LORINCZ is an award-winning author, a nationally recognized speaking coach, and a longtime writing instructor. She's also a successful collaborative writer, recently ranked #7 in Amazon's Kindle Biography/ Memoir writers. Holly reached the top #25 overall with her last collaborative nonfiction book *Crown Heights*, based on a major movie and used to launch a publishing imprint within Amazon.

Holly has books published or in production with St. Martin's Press, Skyhorse Publishing, and Benchmark Press. Her first novel, *Smart Mouth*, won the national 2014 Bronze IPPY Award in Fiction and is optioned for a TV series. Besides being a professional writer, Holly has been editing books for over twenty years, working with multiple *New York Times* bestselling authors. She officially established Lorincz Literary Services in 2010. Once a teacher and a debate coach, and before that the editor-in-chief of a literary magazine, she loves working with stories that will help better the world.